THE SECRET TO THE

WITH COPD

CW00642270

A UNIQUE PERSONAL PERSPECTIVE

FROM A MEDICAL PROFESSIONAL

AND A LATE-STAGE PATIENT

BY

RACHEL GARROD. Ph.D MSc.

AND

DAWN LAWSON

IN MEMORY OF PATRICK MOAN

"We are meant not only to live, but to thrive."

Edie Cartwright

THE SECRET TO THRIVING WITH COPD

INTRODUCTION

This book will have two voices, that of a medical professional working in the field of the treatment of Chronic Obstructive Pulmonary Disease, and that of an "end stage" patient with severe emphysema.

More than 65 million people are diagnosed with moderate to severe COPD worldwide. The great majority of them have no idea how to take an effective breath.

~

This book is intended to be an aid that allows you to take part in your healthcare. Please talk to your doctor about your heart before taking on strenuous activity, such as cardio.

The exercises are examples. They are low impact but powerful. You can find your own on YouTube. You know your body. If something hurts, do *not* do that exercise. Do a modified version, or skip it altogether.

Hopefully by the end of this book you will want pulmonary rehabilitation maintenance. Tell your doctor, your state representative, that person you know who knows people.

If enough of us ask for it, maybe they will give it to us.

TABLE OF CONTENTS

DIAGNOSED AS DEAD

(Dawn Lawson)

Most of us have seen films in which a doctor tells someone that they are going to die. The distance a doctor tries to maintain in a doctor/patient relationship wars with human compassion as the doctor delivers devastating news. The patient struggles to remain brave.

Mine did not go like this.

The doctor was angry. "I have never seen so much damage in the lungs of someone so young!"

I was too stunned to try and remain brave.

I got it. I had done it to myself. Making spectacularly bad life choices had been my superpower for much of my life. Smoking was just one more, but that was the one that got me. I had quit years before, but not in time.

The doctor told me that I would not live out the week. When he took a breath, I asked him if there was anything I could do.

He said, "Yes. Put your affairs in order." He then left the room.

Never bad advice for any stage of life, but as a healthcare plan it lacked promise.

Two years into my diagnosis, too weak to walk across a room, a Facebook group took over my healthcare. They told me that there was something I could do.

Pulmonary rehabilitation. Not for eight weeks, or twelve weeks, for good. At least twice a week for however long I wished to remain alive.

Simply put, Pulmonary rehab is targeted exercise and cardio that strengthens your muscles and heart. The stronger your muscles are, the less oxygen they ask for. When you are weak, just keeping your heart beating can leave you breathless.

PULMONARY REHABILITATION – A PERSONAL PERSPECTIVE

(Rachel Garrod)

If I had a penny for every time a patient said "I'm too breathless to exercise," well…. That is the point. Chronic Obstructive Pulmonary Disease (COPD) is a respiratory disease that results in severe breathlessness, fatigue and often panic or anxiety.

The concept of exercise if you are a sufferer, is madness.

The alternative is much, much worse.

Numerous studies have now proven, beyond any credible argument, the benefits of exercise in people with COPD and other respiratory disease. When you are breathless, often with the most minimal amount of movement, sometimes even at rest, being active can seem an impossibility.

That is why pulmonary rehabilitation, a programme of exercise and education, supporting the patient, is at the heart of effective long-term therapy for COPD.

Pulmonary Rehabilitation is a comprehensive approach that enables patients to work at their own level, to progress gradually, and gives them the knowledge and tools to understand their disease - ultimately enabling the patient to better manage the condition and to be more active with less breathlessness.

In this book, Dawn (a patient with severe COPD whose life was literally saved by pulmonary rehabilitation) and I (a physiotherapist with over twenty years' experience in the academic and clinical world of pulmonary rehabilitation) will describe the components of rehabilitation to the reader in a way that is practical, relevant, and meaningful.

With this book the reader will better understand all aspects of their condition. They will learn practical skills that will enable them to cope with their breathlessness, learn how to undertake exercise that will strengthen muscles, bones and relieve breathlessness.

As a result, they will regain control over their disease and find hope in their life.

AFTER THE DIAGNOSIS

(Dawn)

B*eing diagnosed with Chronic Obstructive Pulmonary Disease is often like spinning a wheel on a twisted game show.*

What happens after the diagnosis has as much to do with your insurance and who your doctor is as it does what "stage" you are at.

We are usually given a death sentence. Five years. One year. Mine, five years ago, was less than a week.

Sometimes a pulmonologist will explain a few things. In the U.S., that often does not happen. I moderate the Facebook COPD group that saved my life. Most new members are confused. They blow in a tube once a year and try to figure out when they are going to die. Many of them are in and out of the hospital, feeling powerless over the relentlessness of this disease, and are running out of hope.

No one explained anything to me. They tried to put a hospital bed in my living room and call it done. For the next few years, I saw nurse practitioners every six months who continued not to explain things.

If someone had taken five seconds to tell me how to take an effective breath, the first two years of my diagnosis would have been much different. That first two years was a semi-living, barely breathing nightmare.

Occasionally people will show up to the site with doctors who engage with them, treat them. These people often have good insurance. Sometimes they simply have good doctors. I eventually did see a good doctor who considered me worthy of treatment, but it took four years. By then Facebook had diagnosed me. I told him what they had prescribed, he agreed, and treated me accordingly. Six months later I found a rock star of a nurse practitioner who explained why my sinuses had been swelling shut every night for five years.

An extremely fortunate few will be referred to pulmonary rehabilitation. Again, mostly good insurance in the U.S. They are more proactive in the UK. In the UK they pay attention to studies and consider rehab a valuable tool in the treatment of patients with Chronic Obstructive Pulmonary Disease. In the U.S. rehab is barely considered.

THAT is where the magic happens. Pulmonary rehabilitation. It turned out that ongoing rehab was available in my area, even without good insurance. No one at the PMA mentioned it.

Medicare does not pay for ongoing rehab. The hospital system I am in decided to offer it on their own. That decision was huge on their part.

Most people do not have ongoing rehab available unless they have good insurance. Most people I know do not have good insurance.

I do not know anyone with ongoing rehab available to them but the people who attend my rehab.

I was tired of waiting to die. I Googled COPD incessantly and got inhaler ads.

My housemate Sel is the only reason I am still walking this earth. Sel, and Patrick Moan.

Sel told me to quit messing around on Facebook and look for a support group.

Hmmm. That had not occurred to me.

I punched COPD into Facebook and found my people. They were not sitting around waiting to die. Several of them had gone decades past their death sentences, had found rehab, and were thriving.

Those who did not have ongoing rehab had managed to work it into their lives, the ones who wanted to live.

Facebook educated me about several things.

These people did not know me. Patrick Moan took the time to talk me into asking for a referral to rehab, although I stated repeatedly that I was too weak to exercise.

Patrick would tell me "Quit arguing about it. Just go. See what happens. Or, lay around and die if you want. You have a choice."

I did not know that I had a choice. As far as I knew, I was dying. It was taking longer than expected, but everyone at the PMA kept assuring me that it was just around the corner.

When the PMA turned me down, Patrick took the time to convince me that if I wanted to live, I would find a way in.

The PMA told me I did not qualify for pulmonary rehabilitation. I was "too far gone". They used med-speak, but that is what it came down to.

I reported to Facebook, my doctor by then. They told me "They are wrong. If you can move, you can benefit. Fight for it."

(I often say I am not a real doctor. I only play one on Facebook. I wish that were a joke.)

It was a process. I had no idea that I could argue with medical professionals. I would make an appointment. The PMA would give me various reasons to justify their refusal to make a referral. I would report to Facebook. Patrick, or someone else, would tell me to make another appointment, giving me arguments to unravel whatever the latest reason was.

By this time, several people were chiming in. I was starting to look like one of the people who might be willing to do what it takes to survive this thing.

They finally made an appointment for me with a doctor who was willing to humor me.

I found out how to breathe.

This is the first thing that happened at rehab: I learned how to breathe.

(RACHEL)

Diaphragmatic breathing is the most efficient form of breathing. It allows air to reach the small airways right at the bottom and helps fill all the alveoli. (Get a good lung full of air.) If we breathe shallowly and from the top, air does not fill the entire lungs. Often people with COPD breathe sporadically with a poor rhythm. It can be difficult to use the diaphragm.

Now things get contradictory. On the one hand I'm saying people with COPD cannot use the diaphragm and on the other I'm saying you must! Which is it? To diaphragm or not to diaphragm!

Slow, relaxed diaphragmatic breathing can be performed by almost all patients with COPD, but it needs to be consciously learnt.

Try this now:

Diaphragmatic Breathing with Pursed Lips Exhalation
Sit on your bed or a sofa with your knees half bent (crooked knees)
Relax your shoulders
Place one hand just below your sternum on your tummy and the other on your upper chest.
Let the air come in.
Let your tummy gently rise as the air flows in.
Keep your shoulders relaxed, aim for very little movement at the top of your chest.
Now breathe out, slowly through pursed lips.

Don't let your cheeks puff out just push the air out in a long slow exhalation.

The shortcut for this is "Smell a flower, flicker a candle."

Inhale through your nose, from your belly. Purse your lips and gently blow for twice as long as the inhale.

They give me little oxygen tanks at the PMA that are "pulse" activated, when you inhale it triggers the pulse feature and oxygen is released. For two years, my breath was too shallow to trigger the pulse feature. I had to set the tanks on continuous flow, which empties them out quickly.

There were times in that two years when I could not make it to the bathroom. I would get out of my chair, take a couple of steps, and go down like a redwood tree. No graceful slumping to the floor. Straight from vertical to horizontal. My roommate Sel would hear the "thud", come out and pick me up, and toss me back into my chair. And I would still have to pee.

There were times I could move, when I could get in the car and try to make it to a doctor's appointment downtown. On continuous flow, the little tanks lasted about 40 minutes. I would load the car with little tanks, eyeing the gage on the tanks while I was driving to see if it dipped into red. When they ran out, I would get to the side of the freeway and change them out in a panic. Sometimes I would change them out in a traffic jam. Usually, I would get most of the way there and realize I did not have enough oxygen to go to the appointment and then get home. I would get off the freeway, turn around, and change the tanks out on the way home.

Every time I saw a nurse practitioner (until I got into rehab, they did not waste doctors on me) I asked them why I could not make the little tanks work. Whatever I asked, the answer was the same. "I dunno. Are you comfortable?" I finally asked what "comfortable" meant. No, I was not comfortable. "Turn your oxygen up until you are comfortable."

"How high?"

"As high as you want."

I did not know it until I found the COPD group, but I had been instructed to kill myself.

Hyperoxia. Too much oxygen makes you sleepy and confused, then dead. Sleepy and confused has become a permanent part of my make-up. I tell people that technically, I cease to exist at four in the afternoon.

TEN MINUTES into rehab, I could activate the pulse feature on the little tanks. It was the first miracle in an explosion of miracles.

I recently looked at a Medicare bill. It cost a small fortune, every time I saw one of those nurse practitioners, who answered every question with "I dunno. Are you comfortable?" How much money was spent over that first two years? In rehab, I got more information in ten minutes than I got out of two years' worth of appointments with nurse practitioners.

The last nurse practitioner I saw was worth her weight in gold. I finally saw a good doctor, four years into my diagnosis.

Without rehab, I would not have lived to see them. Not only am I living, but I am also thriving. I am not in and out of the hospital. I am at the dog park.

WHO SHOULD GO TO REHABILITATION? - EVERYONE!

Dawn was told she was too ill to benefit from pulmonary rehabilitation – but how wrong was that!

Dawn chiming in. If you can move, you can benefit. Period.

The UK also claims some people are "too ill" for pulmonary rehabilitation.

It was at Whitechapel hospital that I first heard about pulmonary rehabilitation. At that time, we would give patients with COPD breathing exercises, help them clear their chest of sputum and try and get them to walk about the ward. Sometimes I'd walk with my patients down to the smoking room and leave them there to have a cigarette. That does not happen anymore!

Our patients would walk around a bit, but that was about it. As to advice on going home, we would simply tell them to do what they could, and rest as much as needed. How wrong we were! For so many years we had simply been giving the wrong advice mainly because it was felt that patients with COPD were "too ventilatory limited to achieve sufficient training stimuli." In other words, their lungs were too bad to allow them to do enough cardiovascular training to make a difference.

In one of our weekly physiotherapy training updates we discussed a research paper from Canada that showed that an eight-week training programme, given to patients with COPD who were in a stable condition - that is, not acutely unwell – resulted in improvements in walking distance and reductions in breathlessness. For a physio, research like this is a godsend to us. **Now we could really dig in.**

The very next day I decided to take one of our patients, let's call him Gene, from the ward to the gym and see how he would fare on the exercise bike there. He was over his acute phase of the exacerbation now and on the mend but still very breathless. He'd been taken off oxygen the last few days but I brought it along with me – just in case. As it turned out I didn't need the oxygen. With Gene's agreement I got him to the gym, and we set about adjusting the bike for his height. At that moment two nurses came rushing into the room and insisted I get Gene back to the ward. The consultant had heard I was about to exercise Gene and had determined this was a "pointless and unnecessary".

His patient was to rest and take it easy.

(*A large portion of the medical community still considers exercise pointless and unnecessary.*)

I think things continued in that vein for another year or so, and I became increasingly frustrated as more and more research showed the benefits of what they were calling pulmonary rehabilitation. It seemed research hospitals all over the world were now bringing patients with COPD to the hospital for exercise and education programmes. Admittedly this was initially for patients in the stable state, not those recently admitted to hospital, but our doctors and respiratory specialists were still insisting there was no point in treating patients this way.

I took an extra qualification in respiratory physiology and did my dissertation on pulmonary rehabilitation. There were just over 400 papers on the topic (a quick google scholar search now shows about 1,570,000 results). Most were positive, but we were still being told not to attempt rehabilitation.

I was fuming.

Then, as it if it were meant to be, I saw an advert for a research physiotherapist to help conduct one of the UK's first randomized controlled trials in pulmonary rehabilitation. I applied for the post and remember saying to a friend that surely, I had to be the most qualified physiotherapist in London for that job. I started what became a five-year research post at The London Chest hospital.

House-bound patients

Our research was complicated, in that we decided to look at two different groups of people with COPD: all patients had severe to moderate COPD but some were able to attend an 8-week out-patient rehabilitation programme while others were house-bound. The patients who agreed to come to the hospital for the research were randomly assigned to two groups – exercise and education or education alone.

We had a fancy new gym with super equipment and a lovely teaching room. Patients attended in groups of 8 – 10. The education programme for each out-patient group was identical, meaning that if there were any differences in breathlessness or exercise tolerance it was down to the exercise component.

Some critics had been saying that positive results were not due to the exercise but due to patients learning more about their health and managing their condition better as a result. This was a reasonable argument and one that our research should be able to answer.

Our other group of patients were housebound folk, people whose breathlessness was so bad they could no longer leave the house, even with the help of a taxi (which with our research funding we could provide). We than randomly assigned these house bound patients to two groups, exercise and education or education alone, but in this case it would be provided at home, individually. Rina and I (another physiotherapist) were employed to provide all the rehabilitation and education in a standardised manner, and to visit the patients at home offering the same exercise and/or education as the hospital group received. Except of course, the home folks did not get quite the same. There was no fancy equipment for a start, and because they were house bound, they missed out on the learning that comes from seeing other people with the same condition as yourself.

Our results showed two things. Firstly, for the group exercising as out-patients, the exercise component of rehabilitation was **essential** to achieving improvements in exercise tolerance and breathlessness.

The patients that received education only **felt** a bit better. There were no statistically significant improvements in exercise or breathlessness.

Secondly, our housebound patients, seen individually at home, did not do as well as our out-patient group. For these folks, unable to get to the hospital even with a taxi, there were no changes in exercise tolerance, either in the exercise only group or in the exercise and education. This is why some guidelines argue that "patients can be too ill for rehabilitation." Our home-based programme lacked some of the equipment we had at the hospital. It also lacked the group effect. We cannot tell if it was the severity of the disease or the lack of equipment/ group support. But the research was interpreted as if some people were "too ill" for rehab. Dawn will tell you in no uncertain terms no one is "too ill" for rehab. And I would support that, but research looks at the average effect and not at individual differences, and people are individuals.

Every single one of us has the power to change our outcome.

I know from clinical experience that movement, however little, has a positive effect on breathing and on quality of life.

Do nothing… and well, that will be the outcome. Or worse!

If you can get to an out-patient programme, if you can get to a gym or a community centre, then do so! If you can get out to walk – then that will help. And if you can´t, then start at home, until you can. Because we know it will help- immensely!

Start with a single chair stand. Sit in a chair, cross your arms, stand. That is it. That is the complete exercise.

When I first started rehab, I could do three chair stands. One may be too difficult for some people. No problem. Stack books on the chair – this will make the exercise easier. Stack however many books it takes to go from sitting to standing. When you have mastered this, start removing books.

I now do ten a day. That is a lie. I try to do ten a day. Chair stands make it easier to move about the world.

What´s the reality, too often?

This *is the reason that physiotherapists, respiratory therapists, and exercise physiologists are the heavy lifters in pulmonary medicine.*

They are interested in the person behind the disease. They are not interested in sitting around, tending to sick people. Not that they have anything against tending to sick people. They are invested, though, in helping us improve our health, battle back the disease.

I was under the care of a Pulmonary Medicine center for almost three years before I met a respiratory therapist and learned that I did not know how to breathe.

In the two years before I found my Facebook group my health steadily declined. I was in the active process of dying.

I had so many questions. I Googled COPD incessantly and got inhaler ads.

(We detest those inhaler ads, with the perky music and the promise that if you use this inhaler, you will be hang-gliding and dune buggy racing tomorrow.)

Every six months I would show up to the Pulmonary Medicine Association I was scheduled at, and pepper whoever I saw with questions. This, this, this, and this was happening. Did it have something to do with COPD? What could I do about it?

My nose was a raw, bleeding wound. I could not activate the pulse feature on the little tanks. Sometimes I could walk, other times I would try to take a couple of steps and hit the floor. Hard.

At my appointments I would bring all these things up, clutching a paper towel to catch the blood dripping from my nose. The answer was the same, to every question. "I dunno. Are you comfortable?" They did not even bother to annunciate.

If one of those medical professionals, anywhere along the way, would have said, "I don't know, but I will ask around", those first couple of years would have been a lot less hideous. I almost did not survive them. I would not have survived if I had not found my Facebook group.

Most people with my lung function do not survive. They would survive if a rehab specialist got ahold of them. Existing pulmonary medicine does not focus on rehab.

Decades of research has suggested that pulmonary rehabilitation should be a core component of treatment for COPD.

Not only is rehab not a core component of treatment for COPD, but most COPD patients I meet for the first time have never heard of pulmonary rehabilitation.

Someone did suggest KY Jelly for my nose, a sexual lubricant. I do not know why I balked at buying KY Jelly. I did not want people to think I was having sex. As if the store clerks cared. Several people offered to buy KY Jelly for me, so someone would think they were having sex. KY did not work. The blood washed it right out of my nose.

What did work, eventually, was a humidifier on my concentrator. I did not know they existed. A sixty-nine-cent plastic bottle. They had them there, in the office, while I was dripping blood. I do not know why they did not give me one or enlighten me about them. It may have been because that first pulmonologist wrote "hospice" on my chart.

It finally occurred to me to punch COPD into the search bar on Facebook. I found my people.

They asked how many liters of oxygen I was on. I told them "I don't know. I just turned the machine all the way up."

"What in the h*** did you do that for?"

"They told me to, at the PMA."

"What is your saturation?"

"What does that mean?"

"Do you have a pulse ox?"

"What's a pulse ox?"

They posted a picture. Oh! The thing they put on your finger!

Saturation – what it is and how to monitor it. Your oxygen saturation is the percentage of oxygen moving through your

bloodstream. You measure it with a pulse oximeter, the thing they put on your finger at the doctor's. They are available on Amazon and at most drug stores for around twenty-five American dollars.

Ideally, you want to keep your saturation between 92-96. Too much oxygen is as bad as not enough – do not turn your oxygen up without consulting your doctor. Yale Medicine says that anything under 90 is considered an emergency. I was taught that 88 is okay, but I am more comfortable at 90. Under 88, it takes about five minutes for brain cells to begin dying.

Ask your pulmonologist for an overnight wristband test to find out what is happening with your saturation while you sleep. This is important. Your body could be struggling while you are asleep.

They told me to turn the machine down, NOW. They explained about too much oxygen, the sleepy, confused, dead thing. CO_2 poisoning. Sleepy and confused has become a permanent struggle, but I did not reach dead.

They told me to get into pulmonary rehabilitation if I wanted to live.

I looked at my dogs. I take in abandoned senior dogs. I needed to outlive my dogs.

I called the PMA and asked if rehab was available. I was surprised when they told me it was. I thought surely someone would have mentioned it in those first couple of years. I told them that I wanted a referral, and they made an appointment.

I was scheduled with a nurse practitioner. (They seldom wasted doctors on me.) He told me "A doctor would have to give you a referral, but you won't get one. You don't qualify."

"What do you mean I don't qualify?"

"You do not have the lung function to benefit from pulmonary rehabilitation."

I heard those exact words, two more times, once after I had been in rehab for over a year and was thriving. It is what they were trained to say to people with low lung function. The last gentleman was hostile – he acted as if I was trying to steal medical equipment.

I reported back to Facebook. My first Facebook doctor, Patrick, told me "They are wrong. Fight for it."

I did have to fight for it. At the time, I would stop and wonder occasionally what I was fighting for. I heard words like "exercise", and even worse, "weights". Exercise did not sound like anything that I wanted to deal with. The less you move, the less you want to move, and by that time I was essentially living in a recliner.

Weights? I could picture myself dropping weights on my foot, or maybe going down and knocking myself out on a barbell. I could see the doctors shaking their heads and saying, "This is why we do not send these people to rehab."

They finally scheduled me with a doctor willing to humor me, and I got on the waiting list.

I had grown accustomed to trying to defend my existence to doctors. When they got out their stethoscopes, I said "You will not hear breath sounds. That does not mean I am dead."

The doctor I was seeing at the time was a nice man, and he had knowledge, but he was tired and ready to retire. I was a bewildering aberration. He tried to describe my lungs to me. He said, "Your lungs…" he fumbled for words, gave up, waved his hands in the air "…are not there." How on earth could I still be walking around with no lungs?

While I was waiting to see if the weights would indeed be a disaster, I asked him if there was a way to find out how long I really had to live. He tried hard to find out. He sent me to a panel of experts at UC San Francisco.

When I met with him afterwards, I asked "How long?"

He looked down at the floor for a moment, then looked up and held up one finger.

I said, "One year?"

"Maybe" he emphasized. He did not think I was going to make it a year.

This was a doctor who cared enough to know this was not good news.

At rehab I expected more of the same.

They greeted me cheerfully, which was a surprise. The best I could hope for with everyone else I had seen was condescending.

People were walking around joking and laughing. I saw the dreaded weights, which turned out to be small and brightly colored. They brought me into the main office, and a doctor pulled out his stethoscope. I said "You will not hear breath sounds. That does not mean I am dead." They laughed. No one had ever laughed.

A senior German Shepherd who had come to live with me had decided that she was an alert dog. She spent her first nine years in a cage as a breeder. When Tasha moved in, she carried the remote control for the television around for two days. She had never had a toy. I let her have it, even though she kept changing the television channels.

Dogs that alert on health distress are rarely trained – they either have it or they do not. It is often rescue dogs, who are grateful and extremely focused on the person who finally shows them love. Tasha knew when my oxygen saturation fell dangerously low before I did. My friends learned to look at Tasha when they wanted to know if I was okay. I lie.

Your brain is the organ that uses the most oxygen, and the organ that suffers first when you lack oxygen. When my saturation dropped, I quickly became too confused to notice that I was confused. Tasha noticed. I do not know why. Doctors have speculated that she smells the CO_2 that rises when your oxygen saturation drops. Whatever it is she noticed, she threw a fit until I noticed, and fixed whatever the problem was.

In a store once, I thought that she urgently wanted to shoplift. It turned out that my portable had frozen up. I got out to the car and on the emergency tank just as things started going black.

Tasha dozed on the floor while they evaluated me for rehab. The doctor put the stethoscope to my back and asked me to exhale sharply. On the sharp exhale Tasha sprang to her feet, lowered her head, and stared hard to see if I was in distress. Or smelled hard. Satisfied that I was not in trouble, she gave the doctor a skeptical look and curled up on the floor again.

"The dog passed!" someone said, and everyone laughed. Laughter turned out to be a strong component of rehab.

As I said, pulmonary rehab was an explosion of miracles.

They told me that I did not have an expiration date stamped on my foot. They answered my questions. If they did not have an answer, they told me that they would find one.

Those three women not only brought me back from the dead, but they also taught me to thrive.

One of the measures they use to define how damaged you are is "tolerance to exercise".

Does it not follow that if you increase your tolerance to exercise, you will find yourself less damaged?

I went from a barely moving, barely breathing existence to a life I consider full and rich. I was diagnosed at 18 percent lung function. After two years of rehab, my lung function measured 24 percent.

Yes, there is a magic pill to battle this thing back with. Movement. Small, targeted exercises in a safe setting.

Many people reading this are now thinking "You are out of your mind. I cannot walk across the room."

It is devastatingly simple. Your muscles require oxygen to move. The weaker they are, the more oxygen they ask for. When I was diagnosed, I stopped moving. I did not feel like moving. The less I moved, the weaker I became.

When you become physically weak, just keeping your heart pumping can leave you breathless.

This whole process of becoming weak? It is reversible. What you feed grows.

When exercising, always have a chair with you. If it hurts, STOP. Do not do that one or do a modified version.

There are a lot of COPD exercises on YouTube. We fill put a few in this book. Find the ones you like, and do a few of them every day, or every couple of days. Put some music on.

Or push yourself a bit harder to do physical things. Dance. Alligator wrestle. The point is **move.**

Pull your shoulders back with your elbows. Hold for a moment. It opens your airways. Tell me that does not feel good.

Do a few shoulder rolls.

You are taking a step towards improving your health.

That is powerful.

REHABILITATION EXPLAINED

Sometimes I think the term pulmonary rehabilitation is all wrong, the implication is that we are somehow providing "rehabilitation of the lungs" – it makes it sound like we can somehow restore the lungs to their previous function. It might also explain why, when I start to teach a patient leg exercises, they look at me as if I'm mad.

"But it's my lungs that don't work, not my legs" they say, understandably.

It is true. The lungs are damaged and much, if not all, of that damage is irreparable.

What are the benefits of pulmonary rehabilitation?

The following is a list of the proven benefits of rehabilitation (countless randomised controlled trials have shown these benefits and the evidence is considered to be "Grade A" – the best evidence:

- Improvements in breathlessness
- Increased exercise tolerance
- Reduced anxiety
- Fewer days spent in hospital due to exacerbations
- Improved quality of life
- Increased peripheral muscle strength

Pulmonary rehabilitation is **cost effective** – a relatively cheap and non-invasive treatment that ultimately saves hospital costs and improves quality of life. So why isn't it available everywhere? Why indeed?

How does it work?

"I can't breathe, my lungs are damaged, how can exercise help?"

This is such a fair comment and one I always try to address the first time I meet a new patient. Yes, your lungs are damaged, catastrophically so in some cases. Being able to breathe is not just down to the lungs.

Sure, the lungs do the clever bit, extracting the oxygen and expelling the carbon dioxide. The body is a whole system, though, not just separate organs.

Take our muscles. The stronger our muscles are the more efficiently they use oxygen. Even with the same amount of oxygen coming into my blood stream, if I have strong legs and arms, I will be able to do more than if my body is weak.

Research has shown that in as much as 40% of people with COPD the main limiting factor to exercise tolerance is muscle fatigue rather than the lung abnormalities.

That part is important. We think that the "not being able to breathe" thing is the problem. In my case, and in the case of everyone else I know who has started exercising, it is muscle strength that turns out to be the culprit.

Similarly, the heart is super important. The heart is a muscle, just as the muscles in your thighs are. It needs to work hard to keep strong. The stronger the heart, the more effectively it pumps blood around the body. After a period of training -- this applies to people with COPD and with heart failure -- the heart rate is lower for a given amount of exercise than it was before the training. If the heart rate is lower, the breathing rate will also be lower. Let us say, today I can walk for 5 minutes at 5 km an hour and my heart rate is 100 beats per minute. After a period of training, I would be able to do that same exercise with a lower heart rate, sometimes as much as 10% lower.

That means my breathing rate will be lower – and if I have COPD, that means I am less breathless!

Improvements in mechanical efficiency also contribute to the improvements seen after rehab. By that I mean the joints and the skeletal structure. If you are stooped and bent because of fear and pain your walking will be hindered, your breathing affected. Teaching postural exercises, joint mobility and stretching helps the body move more freely, in turn making you less breathless.

Another strange mechanism of effect in rehabilitation is something called "desensitisation to dyspnoea".

What this refers to is the brain's response to being breathless (dyspnoea).

(You lose your fear of breathlessness.)

When you have COPD, breathlessness is distressing and frightening.

The panic areas in the brain become extremely sensitive and a negative feedback loop occurs, "I'm breathless, this is scary, I'm more breathless…" and so on. By becoming breathless in a controlled environment, and as a direct result of exercise, the brain becomes a little more resilient to the sensation of breathlessness. There is a desensitisation of dyspnoea.

(Fear of breathlessness can become a self-fulfilling prophecy. Your fear calls your attention to breathlessness, and panic sets in. Panic can cause yet more breathlessness. They feed off one another. Lose the fear and you "magically" become less breathless.)

You can see this with functional MRI scans. The areas associated with fear and panic have less blood flow to them (and therefore less active) after rehab than before.

How we breathe matters also. As part of rehabilitation, we teach breathing exercises like those above. We teach calm breathing and pursed lips breathing for exercise and we help you understand the importance using the diaphragm. Calming breaths can help with anxiety. Rehab teaches all of this, along with a better understanding of the disease and its treatments, these things all contribute to the benefits seen with a pulmonary rehabilitation programme.

One of my patients, recently, took some convincing. He had previously been a good golfer and an active man. COPD had made that increasingly harder. He had stopped golfing, he had also stopped going out, unless it was in the car. Walking made him breathless, so understandably he didn't want to do it. None of the doctors bothered to explain that by doing less he would also become increasingly weak.

His heart would grow weaker, his leg and breathing muscles would waste a little. Over time the breathing got worse. He put it down to his COPD; took more medications and did less. He got heavier. His breathing became increasingly difficult and now it was accompanied by fear and anxiety. By the time I met him, except for walking around the house, he was inactive. This chap, let's call him Jack, had a treadmill in his home. He wouldn't use it. Why would he? His lungs were damaged, how could a treadmill fix that?

We started with a one-minute slow walking on the treadmill. Jack's oxygen levels were low, but not dangerously so, and he got his breath back quickly. One- minute walk, one-minute rest. We also did some work on breathing control. How you breathe, shallowly or deeply, from the tummy or from the top, can make a big difference to how the breathlessness feels. And we did some strength training, in a chair, for those leg muscles.

Over about a period of 12 weeks, Jack did increase his exercise tolerance. His wife noticed a big difference in his breathing around the home and the anxiety was easier to manage. He played golf again, albeit using a buggy and not walking the course, but he was out again. He was able to do 10 minutes continuously on the treadmill. Jack was not going to be cured, but he could breathe again, could move again, and do things. He began to thrive.

Dawn thrives because of her exercises. She does them daily and keeps up the routine. Jack found it difficult to keep up his routine and the golf was gone again.

Pulmonary rehabilitation works. It helps you to improve and thrive. But it is a long-term treatment. **Inactivity is the real killer**. We always tell patients to find something they love doing and keep doing it.

When I worked in London, a couple came to our rehabilitation class, Alice and Mike loved to do "tea dances". Twice a week they joined others at a community centre for an hour's dancing and socialising. But Alice, who was diagnosed with COPD seven years before, was finding it increasingly difficult to manage the dancing. She found she tired more easily and needed to rest more frequently. Her breathing was more laboured, and she felt a bit panicky at times. They thought about stopping the sessions.

Fortunately, they had a good general practitioner (in the UK most people are managed by the local doctor rather than a specialist) so they spoke to him. He referred them to our gym based pulmonary rehabilitation programme.

Alice's aim was to get back to dancing twice a week with Mike. She worked hard on the stationary bike, walking on the treadmill, leg exercises and back exercises. She chatted with the other patients and found what worked for them. She practiced pursed lips breathing and deep tummy breathing. When Alice graduated from pulmonary rehabilitation, she joined a gym with dedicated sessions for older people and she sent us a photo of her and Mike back to waltzing around the room!

Pulmonary rehabilitation works but do what you love.

Pulmonary rehabilitation will work whether you "believe" in it or not. It is not a miracle cure that will work only if you really, really "believe" it will work.

I had friends with cancer who spent a fortune on alternative medicine, who were told it would work if they believed hard enough. When faced with death, they were stunned. They thought it was their fault. They did not "believe" hard enough.

One of the problems we deal with in our Facebook group is predators who try to join under false pretences, then try to sell "miracle cures". They are quickly escorted to the airlock, after I go all evil on them.

There is no cure for COPD. That is the take-home that most patients are left with.

*COPD is one of the few chronic illnesses that you **can** get a grip on, though.*

You can learn to manage and often improve your condition.

When I was diagnosed and told I was going to die, I went straight back to the hospital, where my dad was fighting a losing battle for his life.

I told him I had COPD.

He said, "They can cure that, right?"

I told him "Yeah." In my head – "No."

I got weak. I was sick. I was dying. I did not feel like moving.

The less I moved, the less I wanted to move. The less I moved, the less I was **able** to move.

I looked at the weakness as proof that I was damaged.

I had no idea that I was allowing myself to become weak by laying in my recliner.

What was happening was that through inactivity, my muscles were getting weaker, requiring more oxygen to move them. As I said, just keeping your heart pumping when you are out of shape can leave you breathless.

There are diseases that have their way with you, leave you no say in the matter. My friends who lost their battles with cancer could not have tried harder.

COPD is not one of those diseases. Most COPD patients hold their fate in their own hands.

Most COPD patients in the United States are not given this piece of information.

I finally grew bored, waiting to die. I wondered if I was dying properly. I am a reader. I thought that maybe I should get a book about dying.

I looked around a bit and was not happy with the books I found. They seemed trite, as though I should hire a violinist to accompany me while I read. I finally came across **The End of Your Life Book Club** by Will Schwalbe. It sounded perfect.

It was perfect. It turned out to be a book about living while you are alive.

I was not having fun. More importantly, my dogs were not having any fun. There have been several turning points in my life in which I did things for the dogs that I could not do for me.

They would lose me. I had to think about that, and it did not bear thinking about.

The dogs do not know that they have Will Schwalbe to thank for the dog park. The dogs I had then, the dogs I have now.

My AA sponsor had told me at one point that if I stuck around, I would learn the reason for my existence. I did. I live to make a dog's last days good ones.

I take in abandoned senior and hospice dogs. The first dog that I "permanently fostered" was a Golden Retriever named Mulligan.

Mulligan could have slept anywhere the first night he was here. He chose a spot on the floor in front of my recliner. I grabbed a pillow and blanket and slept next to him. It was his first night here, and I did not want him to be scared.

Mulligan made happy chuffs and snuggled up to me when I put my arm around him.

When I awoke it was to find out he had passed in the night.

I freaked. I thought I had somehow managed to kill the dog. The rescue president told me that is not uncommon. A dog feels safe, and feels it is okay to let go.

*It means **everything** to me that Mulligan died with my arm around him, knowing that he was loved.*

I know that my time with them is limited. Every single dog has healed something that I did not know was wounded or lit something up inside of me that I did not know was there.

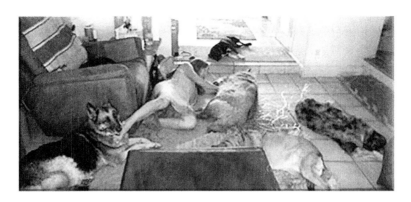

My old superpower was making spectacularly bad life choices. My new one seems to be drawing fortitude from my pack.

I could not find anything on the internet that told me what I could do about my illness, other than "BUY THIS INHALER"! You got the four stages, and the inhaler ads. My lung function was so low that I did not even have a stage. They called it "very end stage".

"End stage" is rarely a thing with COPD. It means that there is nothing more that can be done to improve your condition.

I improve my condition every time I exercise. Not only that, but they also keep inventing new devices. More on that later.

I punched COPD into Facebook and found my people.

I dove headfirst into the group, saying "They told me I was going to die and there was nothing I could do. Is there anything I can do?"

When Patrick told me about rehab, I thought he was out of his mind. He did not understand.

Patrick took the time to argue with me until I gave in and went to rehab.

For two years I had existed in a place that I did not understand. I was dying. I was not dying. My body was doing awful things, and I never knew what or when the next awful thing would be. Sometimes I could walk. Other times, I would crawl to the bathroom, or make my way across a parking lot in stages.

My friend Glenda drove me to a 12 Step meeting once a week. Other than that, I eventually got to the point where I just moved into the recliner. I would hang onto walls to go feed the dogs or try to make the dreaded bathroom trip.

I tried to go small periods of time without the oxygen at first. My friend Lynell asked me at a meeting "Where is your oxygen?"

I told her "I don't want to look like an invalid."

"Oh yes." she said. "That grey half-dead look is much better."

I quit going without the oxygen.

I could care less how it looks now. Sel says I look like Dora the Explorer with the purple backpack.

The cannula gets ripped off my face by some dog flying by at the dog park frequently. Everyone freaks. I just laugh, wipe it down, and put it back on.

I rented a portable oxygen concentrator to fly from California to Florida for a once-in-a-lifetime family reunion. Forty-five minutes into the flight, the portable quit working.

When I got to Florida, I was long past the ability to walk. I paid someone to toss me in a wheelchair and get me to a rental car, where I could plug the portable into a cigarette lighter.

I called the oxygen company when I got to the motel. They told me that the batteries probably had not been charged.

(If you travel anywhere, test the equipment beforehand for however long you are planning on using it.)

I charged batteries all night and went to the reunion the next day. The portable quit working after forty-five minutes.

I did see my Aunt Ann. She introduced herself to me five times. Every time I walked past her, she warmly grasped my hand and said "Hello. I'm Ann. Who are you?"

Aunt Ann was precious.

The oxygen company, not so much.

It was Saturday. If you want to breathe Monday through Friday Eastern Standard Time you are good. Anything outside of those hours, you are on your own.

I spent Saturday and Sunday frantically trying to get a working portable for the flight home at dark-thirty Monday morning.

No luck.

To top the whole thing off, the oxygen company's idea of a portable was a full-sized concentrator on wheels. One of the wheels came off at the Florida airport. A security person stopped the entire line and chased the wheel down, glaring at me as she tested it for explosives.

When she was satisfied that it was a non-exploding wheel, she let me drag the broken portable that now had one wheel to my gate.

I moved as little as possible on the nine-hour trip back to California. I saved fifteen minutes of oxygen to get off the plane. It was almost enough. I passed out at the luggage carousel.

They would not let Sel park outside of the Sacramento airport, but he managed to toss a little oxygen tank inside. I came to breathing oxygen, so someone must have known how to turn it on.

I immediately ordered on Inogen 3, a portable concentrator that fits in my backpack. They let me make payments.

(If you buy your own portable, get the lifetime warranty. It is worth the money.)

For reasons I will never understand, there was no handicapped parking close to the Pulmonary Medical Associates that I was going to at the time. They have a shuttle, but they did not get around to telling me that until just before my doctor retired and I went to a new office. I rode the shuttle twice. Tasha loved it. Living in a cage for nine years had not been kind to her joints.

I would find a parking spot, and we would begin the long trek to the building. When I felt my legs giving out, I would try to make it to a spot where we would not be run over.

*Then the waiting room, and finally the nurse practitioner. Clutching paper towels to catch the blood that constantly dripped from my nose. Every time I went, I would hope that this would be the time they would **talk** to me.*

I might as well have stayed home and questioned a Magic Eight Ball.

I had so many questions. There was the raw bleeding wound that my nose had become. Surely, they had figured out a way to deal with that, had they not? Why could I not activate the pulse feature on the little tanks? If I did manage to make it out, I never knew when my bladder would just decide it was done. That was a special kind of horror. Did that have something to do with COPD?

"I dunno. Are you comfortable?"

"No. I am not comfortable."

"Turn your oxygen up. So you are comfortable."

I tried to do my life. I had made glass paperweights, until I found out that it costs nine hundred dollars a month to generate enough electricity to keep glass molten.

I rented a booth at a Christmas Street Fair in Folsom, California. Once you set your booth up you were stuck there until the Fair ended – the streets were closed. I saved little tanks for months so that I would have enough to make it through six hours on the lowest setting.

I believe it was the unloading of the tanks that undid me. I stood up and tried to get a grip on my breath. My bladder took that moment to quit working.

*I considered not writing about this. Who wants people to know this stuff? Then I thought about people standing in the Bladder Control isle, not knowing **why**, trying to decide between those things and food. Yes, they are that expensive.*

At least it was dark. For six hours I stood in thirty-degree weather and tried to smile at people.

*I asked, every time I went into the pulmonary office. It was on my list of Hideous Things. "Why are these things happening? Do they have something to do with COPD? **What can I do**?"*

"I dunno. Are you comfortable?"

I assume that first doctor put "Palliative Care only" on my chart, "comfort care". Odd that it did not seem to have anything to do with comfort or care. "Palliative Care only" apparently extended to not answering questions. How different would those two years had been if one, just one of those people, had said "I don't know, but I will ask around and get an answer."

Or, if one of them had simply answered questions. I do not think it possible that none of those people had a single answer to anything I asked. I know that they had humidifiers in the room. They left them sitting in the cupboards while I sat in front of them bleeding because the oxygen had dried out my nasal passages.

Turning my oxygen up did not raise my comfort level. It left me brain-addled and exhausted, and it would have killed me if I had not found the COPD group on Facebook in time.

I saved up the little tanks again. I was **going** to make it Downtown to see the doctor at the clinic I went to. She answered questions.

I had two doctors at that clinic that were absolute rocks stars.

My friend Lynell had talked me into seeing the first one. Doctors were not something I did. I had spent a good portion of my life flipping back and forth from being clean and sober to not being clean and sober. Most doctors are not kind to drug addicts.

I was grey, though, and not making a whole lot of sense. I was skeletal – I could not keep weight on. Everyone kept asking me if I was getting loaded again.

I kept telling them that if I was getting loaded, they would know it. I tended to erupt in newspaper headlines when I got loaded.

Doctor Asher was amazing. No condescension, no judgement. She was warm and engaging and thorough. She put the thing on my finger and said "Holy cr*p. You need oxygen." Doctor Asher made things happen. She had me sitting in a pulmonologist's office later that afternoon.

(They did the whole bit of screaming for emergency oxygen, doing their tests, telling me I would be dead within a week, then taking the oxygen away and sending me home.)

Doctor Asher had moved on, but Doctor Montero was also warm, engaging, and thorough. At one point I asked her if she gave trigger point injections – I have a herniated disc that wreaks havoc on my neck and shoulders. She told me she did not. By the next time I saw her, she had taught herself how to give trigger point injections.

Going to an appointment with Doctor Montero was like sitting down in the kitchen of a good friend and working things out.

I asked her if she had any idea what was up with the bladder thing.

She said "That is a common COPD symptom. When your oxygen saturation drops your body shuts down inessential organs to protect the brain and the heart."

Ahhh.

Did they seriously now know this at the PMA? Should you not at least take a token interest in the field of health you are working in? Or was it the "no questions answered" policy?

By the time she had finished the sentence she had sent a script out. She, also, made things happen. Most insurance, even Medi/Medi, pays for those hideously expensive products.

I had, by that time, found the COPD group that continues to save my life on a daily basis. They had given me the miracle of humidifiers, and Ayr, an inexpensive gel. My nose was not a raw bleeding wound any longer. They had taught me what "saturation" meant, and how to monitor it. I was on the waiting list for rehab.

Doctor Montero batted clean-up and fixed most everything else. If it had occurred to me to ask her why I could not activate the pulse feature on the little tanks, she probably would have explained pursed lip breathing. If she did not know it at that appointment, she would have gone home and figured it out.

Once I knew why it happened, I was able to pace myself and make it quit happening. Thanks to Doctor Montero, everyone in the COPD group has access to a Tricks and Hacks sheet that explains inessential organs.

That is one of the benefits of a group. One of us learns something, and we all learn it.

I work in dog rescue, and get phone calls every week from people who want to give up their dogs.

I got a phone call that was a bit different than the usual "The new house does not take pets."

A woman was frantically trying to make plans for her beloved dogs because she was dying. I asked her if she had got a sudden diagnosis. No, she had COPD, but was in the upper stages. I asked her if she knew her lung function. It was three times what mine is.

I asked her why she believed she was dying. Had a doctor told her that? They do that sometimes, I told her.

After circling around it for some time, she told me she was losing control of her bladder. She had asked her pulmonologist if it was COPD related. He told her no and said something about the aging process in women.

She was in her forties.

She told me that she had read that you lose control of bodily functions when you die. That is where her mind took her.

I asked her if it happened when she was out of breath. Yes. I explained about the inessential organ, how your body protects your mind and your heart by deciding that your bladder is not essential.

She cried.

How incredibly sad is that?

This woman had been unravelling her life, giving away her most precious possessions, convinced that her grave was around the corner. It took a faceless dog rescue person to tell her that she was not in the process of dying, that she simply needed to learn to pace herself.

I asked her if she had been to pulmonary rehab. She did not know what that was.

I spent twenty minutes on the phone with her and gave her more information than she had received from several years' worth of doctors and nurse practitioners. She did not know about Ayr. She did not know about mucus relief tablets, and the importance of staying hydrated to deal with mucus. She did not know how to use a nasal spray. Like me before I found out there is a technique to using them, she thought they did not work. She was addicted to Sudafed and did not know that she was addicted to Sudafed. She did not know that Arm and Hammer makes a great non-medicated saline spray with eucalyptus, a natural decongestant.

If she makes it to rehab, she will continuously learn things that will allow her to thrive. Not just live but thrive.

The people who work in pulmonary rehabilitation are an entirely different type of creature than those in medical practice. They want to engage. They want to see us thrive.

She also did not know that a dog's prostate grows differently than in a human, and that in many cases an unneutered dog's prostate will squeeze the urethra shut. She had an older unneutered dog that could barely walk and did not seem to be able to pee. That is something else, though. She now has my vet's phone number. Her vet should have known that.

Working in dog rescue over the years, I have found that some veterinarians close their minds to new research at some point. Although it has been soundly proven that a female dog who goes through two heats is at a 30 percent higher risk of malignant mammary tumors, some veterinarians will suggest waiting a year before altering a dog. They give different reasons, most of which have been disproven.

There is some evidence that early altering can affect bone density in extremely large breeds. I have never known a dog to spontaneously break a bone. I have known plenty of dogs who have died of mammary cancer.

It seems to be the same with pulmonologists. The second pulmonologist I saw designed the rehab program I am in, but he did not believe it would benefit those of us in the lower stages. He knew next to nothing about CO_2. He was an incredibly knowledgeable man, but he stopped looking at research somewhere along the way.

It is difficult, revisiting that first two years after my diagnosis. It was a long painful blur that I try not to think about.

How many other people are existing in that same painful blur?

BREATHING TECHNIQUES AND BREATHLESSNESS

How can breathing techniques work?

Let's talk about Pursed Lips Breathing for a moment – or as Dawn says, "smell a flower, flicker a candle". Pursed lips breathing is magic, literally magic. Many years after I qualified, I ended up teaching Physiotherapy at St George's University, School of rehabilitation Sciences. By this time, I had successfully completed my Doctorate in pulmonary rehabilitation, and I was working as an academic respiratory physiotherapist doing research and teaching. With my first-year students I would bring a patient with COPD in for the afternoon to tell these aspiring physiotherapists what it is like to live with COPD.

Henry was incredible. Like Dawn, he long outlived the expectations of all the medical professionals. He was also funny, charming, and articulate. One student asked him to tell them one thing he had learnt from attending pulmonary rehabilitation. He had laughed and said "There's so many! But one thing sticks out and that was when I learnt how to do pursed lips breathing."

That surprised me because at that time in the UK we, as physiotherapists did not teach pursed lips breathing as it was felt that patients would naturally adopt it if helpful. I asked Henry who had taught him the technique. He told me another patient had shown him. As an aside, one of the hidden benefits of rehabilitation is meeting other people with a lung condition like your own. The comradery can be extremely beneficial. Those of you who have joined a Facebook page COPD Support Group will know that this applies in the virtual world also.

Henry's comment had got me thinking. There had always been a bit of a stand-off between respiratory physiotherapists and respiratory nurses in the UK with regards to the question of pursed lips breathing. We liked to think ourselves the authority on breathing techniques and we just *knew* it was only beneficial to some patients, and those patients would naturally adopt it. There was no point teaching it to non- pursed lip breathers. In fact, we did not know. No one did. There was little research on the topic, and none that addressed the question of who might benefit.

We did a study. I got ethics, always a tedious process but necessary, and engaged some of the students on a "research placement" – I was quite proud of that idea- suddenly I had free research assistants and the students were exposed to clinical research in a friendly environment.

I decided that we needed to test its effects in people with COPD who were not naturally spontaneous pursed lips breathers, so the first part of the study involved asking patients to perform a walking test breathing however they felt most comfortable. Fifteen patients were excluded after this initial test as they adopted pursed lips breathing, that left 54 for the next stage. We then asked them to perform a further two repeatable walking tests in a random order, once breathing normally and once using pursed lips breathing.

We found that a person's walking distance was not affected by whichever type of breathing they used, nor did it affect their breathlessness (as rated by them) at the end of the walk. However, the pursed lips breathing did help reduce the breathing rate at the end of the walk and importantly their breathing recovered back to normal more quickly. On average they returned to normal 6 seconds faster than if they breathed without pursed lips.

I think that's quite a long time if you're gasping for breath don't you?

We were also able to show that those who had the best result from the breathing techniques were those who were most breathless at rest. What is great about this simple piece of research is that we were, for the first time, able to get some real information in clinical guidelines about pursed lips breathing and were able to give proper evidenced based advice to patients. That is the kind of advice I like!

Garrod R., Dallimore, K., Cook, J., Davies, V., & Quade, K. (2005). An evaluation of the acute impact of pursed lips breathing on walking distance in nonspontaneous pursed lips breathing chronic obstructive pulmonary disease patients. Chronic Respiratory Disease, 67–72. https://doi.org/10.1191/1479972305cd068oa

Pursed lip breathing never occurred to me. It was counterintuitive. My breath was so shallow that I panicked a bit every time I exhaled. I felt as if precious breath was escaping.

A good exhale is crucial for a good inhale. As a result of subconsciously refusing to exhale, my inhale was shallow. Nothing out, nothing in. It took me a few minutes to purse my lips and let my breath escape on purpose. Once I did that, though, there was room for a deep inhale. It was the first deep breath I had taken in years.

Yes, it is magic.

BREATHING

This might be a good time to explain how the air gets into our lungs. People sometimes think that we "suck air in", but that's not the case. Air simply flows into our lungs due to changes in to pressure within the chest cavity.

I will explain. Those little receptors in the brain are in fact balls of specialised cells that detect when CO_2 levels rise and trigger impulses to initiate contraction of the muscles of respiration. We have several muscles involved in respiration, but the main one is the diaphragm. This is a big dome like structure that sits just underneath the lungs and above the abdomen. The top part of the diaphragm is thickened connective tissue that merges with the bottom of the lungs. When the diaphragm contracts it flattens and moves lower down. This pushes the tummy contents out and elongates the thoracic cavity (the area within our ribs and sternum) pulling the lungs down.

We also have intercostal muscles which run along-side our ribs, these contract too and help to lift the rib cage up and out – known as the bucket handle action.

Core exercises will also make these muscles stronger, which aids in breathing.

These muscle contractions mean that the volume inside the chest and the lungs is now bigger. This drops the pressure within the lungs, making the air pressure **outside** our lungs higher compared to **inside** so air flows in.

Once you understand this you can see why it is so important to use our diaphragm during breathing.

For some people with COPD this can be hard. It is also difficult to breathe correctly if the person is overweight. The diaphragm may have been pushed upwards into an inefficient position by a swollen tummy.

*Exercising your core muscles will help you keep your stomach under control, making it easier to breathe. Core strengthening exercises are simple, and they feel good.*Ideally, we use our nose as the entry point. People sometimes forget that the nose is part of the respiratory system, its design is so perfect that it will moisten and warm the air before it reaches the lungs.

The little hairs in our noses are there to trap particles and bits of debris we don´t want in our lungs, making it another good reason to try to avoid mouth breathing.

Inhaling is essentially a passive process. Of course, we can make it active and engage additional muscles (the ones down the side of the neck sometimes come into operation when breathing heavily). Singing and laughing and talking all require more active breathing than relaxed normal breathing. Imagine the diaphragm is now flat against the stomach, after the initial contraction it relaxes again and moves back upwards to its original dome shaped position. This forces the air out of the chest cavity and the lungs, and we exhale.

Again, we can do this consciously, but most of the time this is an unconscious act, like breathing in.

I had heard "Breathe from your diaphragm". I had a hard time figuring out where my diaphragm was. I know the general area, but I could not feel it. Someone at rehab said something about babies being natural "belly breathers". Ahhh.

"Breathe from your belly."

If you want to practice breathing from your diaphragm, or your belly, lie on the floor and put a book on your belly, under your ribs. Move the book up and down.

Stand in front of a mirror and watch yourself breathe. If your shoulders are moving up and down, you are breathing from your chest, not your diaphragm. You are not getting the crucial exhale and the deep inhale.

Watching testimony in the Derek Chauvin trial, I finally came to understand how the diaphragm works. It is a bellows system!

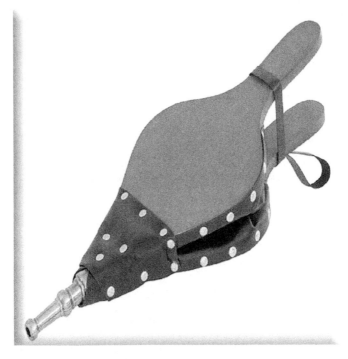

The diaphragm contracts and flattens when you inhale. This creates a vacuum effect that pulls air into the lungs.

If you carry extra weight, it will be harder to fill your lungs. This is why core exercises are important.

The weight of the fat on the chest wall decreases the amount of room for the lungs. It also pushes up on the diaphragm, restricting its movement, particularly when bending over or lying down.

Pursed lip breathing and practicing breathing from the diaphragm, or the belly, will help you fill your lungs.

Why am I breathless?

It is so important to understand the cause of your breathlessness.

Not all breathlessness is equal!

It is especially difficult to understand why you might be breathless if your oxygen levels are relatively normal.

In the absence of measuring oxygen from blood we use something called a pulse oximeter. A pulse ox is a little clip on your finger (or ear). This tells us the percentage of your red blood cells that are saturated with oxygen – normal is 96-98% For COPD normal may be 94-96%. If your oxygen saturation is lower than 92% at rest, it is worth seeing a doctor to determine if oxygen would help you.

The first thing the COPD group taught me when they took over my health care was to measure my saturation. They sent me a link to order a pulse ox off Amazon.

Never start on oxygen without medical advice – it is a drug that can be harmful if not accurately prescribed.

Let us assume your oxygen level is normal – 94% or above. But you are still breathless – why?

Several things will affect breathing in people with COPD.

- Panic and poor breathing techniques can make you breathless - this even happens in people with healthy lungs. See above for some information on breathing techniques.
- Trapped mucus will block airways, causing collapse, making what lung capacity you have less efficient.
- Bronchospasm (where small airways get closed due to muscle spasm) will contribute to breathlessness – your inhalers are designed to help treat this.
- Weak respiratory muscles (especially if you have recently been ventilated), as well as generalized deconditioning will make you more breathless during activity.

The weaker your muscles are, the more oxygen they ask for.

The most common cause of breathlessness in people with COPD is hyperinflation.

Hyperinflation is simply air trapping.

Hyperinflation occurs because of loss of elasticity in alveoli (air-sacs). Instead of being nice and springy, like balloons, the alveoli become floppy and "baggy" like old tights.

This means that the air that should have been squeezed out of the alveoli during expiration gets stuck there. The airways leading to these air sacs shut down and the air is trapped in the lungs.

Parts of the lungs are now filled with deoxygenated air and this air trapping makes it harder to fill the lungs with fresh oxygenated air. When people move around, they naturally need to breathe faster. When this happens the time available to expel air is reduced, making the hyperinflation worse.

This is usually the reason people with COPD find they get so breathless when being active or doing exercise.

The trick to help improve this is breathing to maximise the expelled air- **pursed lips breathing** is great here. Inhalers will help open your airways. Always use your reliever inhaler 20 minutes or so before exercising.

If you use an inhaler with a steroid in it, rinse well and gargle to prevent thrush. Rinsing and gargling with warm salt water is ideal.

The great news is that there is evidence to suggest that a programme of pulmonary rehabilitation may help to reduce air trapping in the long term.

I would be among that evidence. The more I exercise, the less breathless I find myself. When I am moving around, I naturally find myself pursed lip breathing.

Remember the mantra - "When in doubt – breathe out!"

HOW TO BREATHE: THE SEQUEL
CONGESTION

had not been on oxygen long before I became too congested to sleep. I cannot sleep when I cannot breathe through my nose. That was probably [for the good – as I receive oxygen through a nasal cannula, I might not have woken up.

I was miserable. I tried everything I could find over the counter, often all at the same time. I could breathe while I was awake, but every time I relaxed and closed my eyes, I became congested.

I called the PMA. They told me to get Flonase. I got Flonase. It did not help.

I called the PMA again. They said they would talk to a doctor and call me back. After two more sleepless nights and no phone call, I called them. They told me that the doctor said that I would not be scheduled for a stuffy nose and asked me to stop calling them.

I called my medical clinic in the middle of one miserable night. I was going to leave a message. A live person answered the phone. I was not prepared for that – I had no idea what to say. I burst into tears and hung up.

A trauma nurse called me back.

She told me I had been taking the wrong things. She told me to take Sudafed, a drug with Pseudoephedrine in it.

I immediately went to an all-night pharmacy and got some. It worked. I got a full night's sleep for the first time in a long time.

I took it without fail for almost five years.

*Do **NOT** do that.*

Drugs containing Pseudoephedrine are like heroin for the sinuses, just as nasal sprays containing Oxymetazoline are heroin for the nose. Pseudoephedrine simply takes longer.

*I learned about a condition called **rebound congestion** with nasal sprays right away. **Never** use a nasal spray that contains Oxymetazoline for more* *than three days in a row. With continued use, these nasal sprays start to cause the problem they are used to relieve. Your nose becomes addicted quickly. They starve the nose of nutrients and oxygen, and your body compensates by enlarging the veins in the nose, causing congestion.*

I have known people who needed surgery to correct damage to the sinuses created by nasal sprays with Oxymetazoline.

It turns out the same rule applies to drugs for congestion containing Pseudoephedrine. Never take them for more than three days in a row. Do not take them at all, if you can help it.

*Fortunately, by the time the Pseudoephedrine got me, my old doctor had retired. I was going to a different PMA in the same system. The doctor and the nurse practitioners who were seeing me were **treating** me.*

The doctor's assistant I spoke with over the phone told me she was surprised they had not put me on an allergy medicine. She said that was usually the first thing they did for patients with congestion.

I did not tell her that they tried to put a hospital bed in my living room and essentially called it done.

She had an allergy medicine prescribed and scheduled me with a nurse practitioner. That nurse practitioner gave me a miracle.

She explained nasal sprays to me.

99% of a nasal spray's effectiveness lies in the technique in which it was used.

You want to get something with a corticosteroid in it, like Flonase. They were correct about the product at the old PMA – I simply did not know how not use it. I snorted it.

That does not work.

Lean forward and aim the spray towards the top of your nose. Sniff gently. Your sinus cavities run under your eyes and into your forehead. Roll your head from side to side, sniffing gently, so the nasal spray can enter your sinus cavities. I briefly turn my head upside down, still sniffing gently. The nurse practitioner did not tell me to do this part, but I do everything I can to get the nasal spray to go where it should and stay there.

I have not been congested since that momentous appointment.

It is crucial to stay hydrated. Caffeinated sodas do not count. When you are dehydrated your sinus passages dry out and swell, making it too difficult to breathe.

When I had pneumonia the first time, I discovered the miracle of sinus rinses.

Being on just this side of death has done me some favors. I did not have the luxury of considering sinus rinses too weird.

The human body produces something like a quart and a half of mucus daily. When pneumonia struck, I felt like the entire quart and a half was packed into my sinuses.

A breath will do you no good if it cannot make its' way to your lungs.

I watched a YouTube video of a three-year-old child performing a sinus rinse. I had no excuse to not get the little squeeze bottle and go for it.

Distilled water only. *Contracting an amoeba infection in your brain because you used tap water would suck.*

People used to do contortions with the Neti Pot, a little teapot, over the sink. This is no longer necessary.

I got the squeeze bottle from the YouTube video, and a wonderful little device called The Sinugator. You push a button, and it shoots water up one nostril and out the other, taking with it stuff you really do not want to look at too closely.

I hung out in the bathroom for two days with The Sinugator and got through pneumonia without being hospitalized. The Sinugator, and Prednisone and antibiotics.

With my lung function, the internet keeps insisting that my next hospitalization will be my last.

Cold water is unpleasant. For an eight-ounce rinse, I microwave it for 30 seconds.

I have moved on to the SinuPulse. It looks like a water pick, and the reservoir holds sixteen ounces of distilled water. It has ten speeds – I go with the highest.

The first time I used the SinuPulse I was stunned. I could breathe. On impulse, I grabbed my peak flow meter. I normally blow one hundred points (not a good score). After using the SinuPulse, I blow **one hundred and fifty points**. That extra fifty points is significant.

For the sixteen-ounce rinse, I microwave a coffee cup full of distilled water for one minute, then fill the rest of the reservoir from the water jug.

They come with little packets of powder to mix in the water. When you run out you can either buy more packets or make your own solution. For an eight-ounce rinse, use one-half teaspoon of non-iridized salt and one-half teaspoon of baking soda. For a sixteen-ounce rinse, use one teaspoon of non-iridized salt and one teaspoon of baking soda.

Keep your equipment clean. I spray everything with rubbing alcohol before and after I use it, including the spoon I use to mix in the solution, the bottom of the reservoir, and the top of the machine the reservoir sits on.

Sinus rinses have been a miracle for me, but if you do not have issues with mucus, it may be best not to use them. Some doctors believe they may strip natural sinus immunities. Other doctors disagree with this finding, saying that another mucus blanket quickly forms. In my experience, I have never found myself short of mucus.

I cannot take a full breath in the morning until I do a sinus rinse. If I do not do one in the evening, I battle mucus at night.

(Since writing this I have received a brand-new device, the Life2000. An extremely portable non-invasive ventilator. I wear it swinging from my waist and get a full breath most of the time now. I have not had to do sinus rinses since I have been using the Life2000. It turns out that a full breath keeps mucus from building up. Who knew?)

I whiled away many Friday nights hanging out with my dogs and happily studying mucus. I have had plenty of wild Friday nights, some of them lasting years. I must now figure out how to deal with the damage I did to my body while I was busy making epically bad life choices.

I have learned is that there are online support groups for people addicted to Afrin. It is no fun being strung out on Afrin. My second doctor was kind enough to put me on a course of Prednisone to wean my off it and told me to never go near it again.

I suppose that I am grateful that I have not been tempted to suffer an Afrin relapse.

I wish someone would have said something about Pseudoephedrine, the active ingredient in Sudafed. It took several days of Googling before I finally saw the dreaded words **rebound congestion.**

Mucus is the human body's flypaper. Fine particulate matter is our enemy. Mucus traps harmful matter before it can get to the lungs. We swallow most mucus, where it is efficiently dealt with by stomach enzymes.

Mucinex, brand-name and generic, is enormously helpful in dealing with stubborn mucus. Only **100% Guaifenesin**, though. They offer "multi-symptom", which has – you guessed it – Pseudoephedrine in it.

If you take a mucus relief product it is crucial to stay hydrated. If you have mucus issues it is crucial to stay hydrated. Every portion of your respiratory system needs moisture to function properly.

Steam is great for relieving congestion. Ironically, many people with COPD have difficulty breathing in steam. Showers can be a nightmare. (More about showers in the Tricks and Hacks Chapter.)

A warm, wet washcloth works well for those of us who do not want to do battle with a shower. Use pursed lip breathing. Place a warm, wet washcloth over your nose, inhale. Take it away, purse your lips, and gently blow. Repeat until you are breathing easier.

I found a humidifier on my oxygen concentrator essential. No one mentioned them, and I suffered for it until I found the COPD group.

Fortunately, it was only painful nose bleeds. I know someone who suffered a collapsed lung as a consequence of not having a humidifier on her concentrator.

I also have a humidifier on my Trilogy. It warms the water, enabling the airflow to bring a lot of moisture with it. The one night I slept without it I woke up in the middle of the night feeling like my nose was on fire.

If your nose needs more moisture, there is an inexpensive gel called Ayr that is sold at most drug stores.

Saline sprays are great. Arm and Hammer makes a non-medicated saline spray with an extra kick, and another one containing eucalyptus, a natural decongestant.

Mucus produced by the rest of the respiratory system, excluding the nasal passages, is called phlegm.

Mucinex (100% Guaifenesin) will also help loosen phlegm. Again, drinking a lot of water is crucial.

Some people find the HUFF method of coughing helpful in bringing phlegm up. Lean forward and say "Hff!" as loud as you can. Huff without the u.

There is also a device you can blow into called the Flutter Device. It combines positive expiratory pressure therapy with high–frequency oscillations within the airway, loosening phlegm. It sounds complicated, but it is just a piece of plastic you blow into.

Respiratory therapists and physiotherapists work with you to explain all of this. The great majority of those with COPD will never see a respiratory therapist or a physiotherapist, and most doctors are not big on explaining things.

So, we find each other. The fortunate few who have rehab available, or doctors who are willing to talk to them, pass on precious bits of knowledge.

One thing you do have to look out for with mucus and phlegm is color. White is good. Yellow is okay, unless it is all yellow all the time. Yellow can just be old. If it is always yellow, or is turning yellowish green, that may be sign of an infection. Call your doctor.

Pink or red means there is blood – call your doctor.

If your doctor tells you that you are not due to come in for another four months, get another doctor.

A visit to the emergency room may be called for. Yes, you are bothering them. They are paid for that. Take hand sanitizer with you, and a sheet, to keep between you and anything you may be sitting on or leaning against. Yes, you will look paranoid. You get to live through your visit to the emergency room. There are sick people there.

Some people in small towns may not have access to another doctor. Find the closest teaching hospital. They stay up on current research.

Brown could mean an extremely persistent infection.

Charcoal or grey could be due to smoking or being around smoke.

***

If you are smoking, you are not doing yourself any favors.

I get it. It is hard.

I spent thirty years "trying" to quit smoking. What I was doing was trying to see how long I could go before I smoked again. I was convinced that I could not quit – I knew that I would smoke again.

Trying to cut down on cigarettes was even worse. My entire existence was laser-focused on when I could have the next cigarette.

It turned out that the hardest part of quitting was to finally make the decision to put them down.

After that, every craving you resist weakens the next craving. Conversely, every cigarette you smoke sets up the next craving. Smoking is a lot like feeding a tapeworm. You resist a craving; you starve the tapeworm and it shrinks to nothing.

We do not give the people in our group who smoke a hard time. They know they need to quit. It is a horrifying addiction. You know what you are doing to yourself. You know you need to quit. You are utterly convinced you cannot.

My biological mother chased me out of the house with an ax when I was fourteen years old. She did me a favor. Living with her was — problematic. My "real" mother, Connie, took me in and helped heal the damage from the biounit.

The woman who grew me up, the mother of my soul, was Grady O'Hara. We spent many hours sitting together and chain smoking.

When Grady was diagnosed with throat cancer, the first question I asked was what I could do for her.

"Quit smoking" was her answer.

I did not quit smoking. I believed that I was not capable of quitting. It turned out that I was unwilling to make the decision to just put the damned things down.

I took it to the wall. I remember crawling down the hallway, choking and gagging, pausing to take a drag off a cigarette.

***Then** I got strung out on e-cigarettes. They were magic. I could smoke in my sleep without setting anything on fire.*

They did hideous damage to my lungs. I saw the visible evidence. A lung scan before and after a year of smoking e-cigarettes. I was stunned. I had believed them harmless. I had written my e-cigarette supplier a letter thanking them for saving my life.

It was right there in front of me, though. Any sign of tissue that had been vaguely healthy was gone, scarred, blackened.

I do not know why e-cigarettes do so much damage. I know the "smoke" (steam) goes into your lungs hotter than regular smoke. I know there are kids on ventilators because of e-cigarettes.

They still do not know the exact cause of the damage. Some of it looks like chemical burns.

Popcorn Lung can result from e-cigarettes, named after a disease first found in workers in popcorn factories that were exposed to butter flavouring. Popcorn lung is an irreversible condition in which the tiny air sacs in the lungs become scarred and constricted. This results in no air movement in the lungs. You basically smother to death. The only treatment for Popcorn Lung is a lung transplant.

A few years ago, I told someone "In ten years' time a lot of people are going to be saying Oops."

It has not taken ten years.

Nearly three thousand cases of "Vaping Disease" have been reported in the U.S., and there have been sixty-eight deaths. These were the statistics in February 2020. Mostly young people.

It is just beginning.

I knew how it went with cigarettes by then. I made the decision and put them down.

***

I was up at 5:30 this morning trying to figure out how phlegm leaves the lungs. (See – isn't this fun?) It is still a mystery to me. I do not have the lung power to cough anything up. Huff coughing and percussive devices do nothing for me. (I called it the Flutter Thingie for years. I knew that was not the Latin term. I did not know how close I was to the real name.)

I gave away the Flutter Device they gave me at rehab, because it did nothing for me. I threw away my peak flow meter because I did not want to know exactly how much I sucked at breathing.

Someone at rehab finally talked me into taking my readings every morning. Saturation, temperature, pulse rate, and peak flow. She said, "If you normally blow 100, and you cannot reach 80, you will know there may be a problem."

*I ordered a peak flow meter from Amazon because I did not want to admit I had thrown mine away. She was good. I blew exactly 100. **Except** after sinus rinses – I gain an extra 50 points for a while. Then mucus slowly starts setting up camp again. As I said, I have never found a shortage of mucus to be a problem.*

I have no coughing power. None. The only time I cough is when I am choking on my Trisquit crackers.

*(Why on **earth** is there no barrier between the air/food and water intakes?)*

*I have no idea where the phlegm in my lungs goes. I **do** know how to make it go – wherever it goes.*

Have I mentioned that a lot of water is crucial? Water. Is. Crucial.

Steam helps. If you are among the group of us who have difficulty breathing in steam, breathing through a warm washcloth over your nose and mouth is helpful. Again, pursed lip breathing.

Warm compresses on your chest can relieve chest congestion.

There are also several things you can drink that relieve chest congestion.

Fresh pineapple juice reduces phlegm, is a natural cough suppressant that is more effective than most commercial cough syrups. Fresh pineapple contains bromelain, a protein-digesting enzyme known for its anti-inflammatory properties. I have been drinking pineapple juice, even though I do not have trouble with coughing (aside from the odd Trisquit incident). After years of telling other people to drink it, I decided to try it. I now find my body craving pineapple juice. Fresh chunks of pineapple work also.

A teaspoon of apple cider vinegar in warm water with some honey helps relieve chest congestion. To my knowledge there have been no official studies on the benefit of apple cider vinegar, but it is the absolute go-to for several people I know in dealing with colds, congestion, or infection. Hippocrates, the father of modern medicine, used vinegar to clean wounds more than 2,000 years ago. There has got to be something to it, and I cannot find any risks if you stick to a teaspoon in a glass of water.

My immune system has gone sideways. I do not like the term "immune compromised". It makes me sound like an escaped laboratory experiment. I periodically deal with infection. Apple cider vinegar has gone on the shopping list.

***That** is the benefit of finding your people. We compare notes. We know our bodies. We know what has worked and what has not worked. When that nurse practitioner explained there was a technique involved in using nasal* sprays, that information immediately went to my people. They, in turn, give me their information. We heal each other.

We all think that we are weird because we cannot stand the shower, until we find each other.

Turmeric and ginger have been reported to help with congestion. Turmeric also helps with inflammation. It is a great supplement if you have COPD.

I accidentally found out that ginger helped me breathe, then later found it on the last of natural congestion relief ingredients.

One of my COPD symptoms is "wasting". I have a hard time keeping weight on. I burn far too many calories trying to breathe, and most food does not appeal to me. It is difficult to force myself to eat. They had the word "anorexic" on my chart at the old PMA. That irritated me to no end. I was not doing it on purpose.

The first couple of years into my diagnosis, size 0 pants hung on me. My housemate Sel is the reason I stopped looking as if I should be hanging from an anatomy hook. He quietly cooked things until he stumbled upon something I would eat. Egg salad was the first thing. Now he has got me addicted to lasagne.

The woman who helps me moderate the COPD group suggested eggnog. I like eggnog. Lots of protein, lots of calories.

I got a little blender. A cup of milk, three eggs, a little sugar, vanilla, cinnamon, ginger.

Scrub the eggs thoroughly before you crack them.

I accidently dumped half a bottle of ginger in the blender once. I removed what I could, but I ended up with eggnog that had far more ginger in it than I would normally use. I took a sip and my sinuses opened.

I now drink ginger with some eggnog in it.

EDIT: Since I have had the Life2020 ventilator I have not been congested. No sinus rinses. No Mucus Relief tablets. With a full breath, mucus does not build up. Who knew?

SHORTNESS OF BREATH

What is the most important muscle in breathing?

The DIAPHRAGM is the most important muscle to breathing.

In fact, the diaphragm has its' own nerve supply and can work involuntarily and voluntarily. The diaphragm works like a vacuum. When the diaphragm contracts during inhalation, it goes down toward the stomach, expands the lungs and pulls new air into them.

During exhalation, the diaphragm relaxes and moves back to its original position. As the diaphragm relaxes, it and the intercostal muscles in the ribcage push old air back out of the lungs. The intercostal muscles also relax and reduce the space in the chest cavity.

Accessory Muscles

If you are under stress, have an injury or are having trouble breathing, accessory muscles can help you breathe. Accessory muscles are not used during normal breathing. The accessory muscles sometimes used from breathing include the muscles in front of the neck, the chest pectorals and the abdominal muscles. For people with COPD, air becomes trapped in the lungs and makes it harder for them to expel air. Many people with chronic lung diseases use accessory muscles to help them breathe in and out.

What is Shortness of Breath? ~~ DYSPNOEA

Shortness of breath is a common and often frightening symptom of chronic lung diseases.

Many people describe breathlessness as air hunger.

Shortness of breath makes people feel like they cannot fill their lungs with oxygen. Sometimes, shortness of breath happens suddenly and without a known cause. It often occurs with chest tightness and anxiety.

If you experience shortness of breath, follow your doctor's instructions and use prescribed inhalers as directed by your doctor. While frightening, remember to stay calm and consider trying the following positions to reduce shortness of breath.

Best Positions to Reduce Shortness of Breath

In combination with the pursed lips breathing and the diaphragmatic breathing techniques, these positions to reduce feelings of shortness of breath can help you relax and reduce the sensation of breathlessness.

Sitting Positions to Reduce Shortness of Breath:

Typically, shortness of breath happens during activity, emotional experiences, bad or changing weather conditions or when you feel tense or stressed. Try these sitting positions to reduce shortness of breath:

SIT HOLDING YOUR CHIN to Reduce Shortness of Breath

Sit in a chair or in a comfortable position

Keep your feet flat on the floor

Lean your chest forward a little

Rest your elbows on your knees

Place your chin in your hands (if you feel comfortable doing so)

Relax your neck and shoulders as much as you can

Practice your breathing techniques

SITTING FORWARD Position to Reduce Shortness of Breath

If a pillow is easily available, place it on a table

Sit in a chair at the table

Keep your feet flat on the floor

Lean your chest forward some

Place your arms on the table

Relax your head on your forearms (if a pillow isn't available) or rest your head on the pillow

Use your breathing techniques

STANDING Positions to Reduce Shortness of Breath:

Sometimes, shortness of breath happens suddenly. If a chair or a place to do the sitting positions isn't available, give a standing position to reduce shortness of breath a try:

Standing Position A:

Find a sturdy wall

Stand with your feet shoulder width apart

Lean your hips on the wall

Let your hands rest on your thighs

Allow your shoulders to relax

Lean forward slightly

Let your arms dangle in front of you

Remember to practice your breathing techniques

Standing Position B:

Find a strong piece of furniture (just below shoulder height), such as a table

Stand at the furniture

Place your elbows or hands on the chosen furniture

Lean forward a little

Relax your neck and shoulders

You can rest your head on your forearms if your elbows are on the furniture

Utilize your breathing techniques

Sleeping Positions to Reduce Shortness of Breath:

If you are at home or are awakened by an episode of shortness of breath, remain calm and consider these sleeping positions to reduce shortness of breath:

Sleeping Position A:

Lie on your Left side

Place a pillow between your knees

Elevate your head with a pillow or two

Keep your back as straight as possible

Relax and use your breathing techniques

Sleeping Position B:

Lie on your back

Place a pillow under your knees, so your knees are bent

Elevate your head with a pillow or two

Allow yourself to relax

Practice your breathing techniques

THE MAKING OF A PULMONARY REHABILITATION PROFESSIONAL

*I*n the US we have respiratory therapists and exercise physiologists. In the UK, they have physiotherapists.

You have noticed by now that we spell words differently on our respective sides of the ocean. As I said, this book is written with two voices. It is written for those with COPD , and those that care for them, all over the globe. Treatment differs drastically. People do not.

Becoming a Physiotherapist

I was thirteen when I decided I wanted to be a Physiotherapist. My mum was having treatment for a frozen shoulder that had occurred after mastectomy for breast cancer, "The shoulder caused more problems than the cancer," she joked. I don't think that was true but she was a stoic woman. Mum's treatment was hydrotherapy-exercises and stretching in warm water. We both got in the heated pool and I splashed around pretending to help. I loved water and as far as I was concerned this was the job for me- I could spend all day in what was effectively a large heated bath.

As it turned out there is a lot more to Physiotherapy than hydrotherapy treatment, but that was good enough for me. Mum got better and I told the careers officer at school my decision. She was less than impressed. "Are you sure? Physiotherapy is very hard to get into; you must be academic. I'm not sure that's you. Perhaps try hairdressing instead?"

Those were her exact words. I'm not sure what she had against hairdressing, but there you go. I took no notice. I've never really cared much for other peoples' opinion of me. So, I applied myself (perhaps the careers officer had a point). I worked hard in the subjects I knew I would need, Biology, Chemistry, Physics, Maths. English was a doddle as I've always loved that, the rest I let go by the wayside. I never learnt any languages. I spent most of my time outside headmaster's office for bad behaviour.

I regret that a little now as I live in Spain and am hopeless at the language.

I ditched Geography after calling the teacher a *stupid old cow,* I muddled through a few other subjects and eventually got the A levels I needed to apply to practice Physiotherapy. After a couple of years doing fun things like working in ski resorts and catering for rock bands on tour – yes really! I did the European leg of The Joshua Tree tour with U2 which as you can imagine was a ball – I started at Guy's School of Physiotherapy, London, UK.

I never intended to specialise in respiratory physiotherapy. I'm not even sure I knew it existed then. My wild living - smoking and drinking a good bit - pretty much ruled out sports physio. I really couldn't get my head around those folks! Neuro Physio, looking after people who have had strokes or other neurological disorders was discounted after I fell whilst on holiday and broke a spinal vertebra. Luckily, I was okay, but neuro physio in those days was tough on the back. And I liked my respiratory patients. They were funny, quirky, stoic – like my mum – and I felt I could relate.

In 1993, I was 24 years old and working at Whitechapel Hospital in London. I had done my junior rotations, and specialised in cardiorespiratory work. I looked after patients on the cardiac wards, delivered cardiac rehabilitation with a great team of nurses. I worked in intensive care units helping folks on ventilators keep their chests clear and I saw patients on the medical wards. Patients with COPD.

In those days we didn't call it COPD. When I was training the disease was called Chronic Airflow Limitation, during my training it was changed to Chronic Obstructive Airways Disease. and patients were given the dreadful medical terminology of "Blue Bloaters" or "Pink Puffers".

Pink Puffers and Blue Bloaters

What awful labels – however they made a bit of sense. Blue Bloaters are patients with COPD who retain CO_2, these patients have chronically low levels of oxygen in their blood – hence the "blue" - and should only be given a limited amount of oxygen as too much may cause them to stop breathing.

Most people imagine we take a breath in because our oxygen levels fall. That would actually be a dangerous way for the body to work. In healthy people oxygen blood levels are always maintained to nearly 100% saturation. Chemoreceptors (a specialised ball of cells) in the brain detect a build-up of CO_2 that occurs as a natural by-product of metabolism. We breathe as a result of stimulation to these chemoreceptors. We breathe in oxygen; it goes to the lungs and then diffuses across thin-walled air sacs (alveoli) into capillaries (small blood vessels). This oxygen rich blood then passes through the pulmonary vein to the right side of the heart, first to the top (the atrium) and then to the bottom (ventricle) where it is squeezed out and travels, via the aorta, to the rest of the body.

On the other hand, blood depleted oxygen travels, via the vena cava, to the left side of the heart. This time, contractions of the heart squeeze the blood through the left atrium to the left ventricle and out through the pulmonary artery back to the lungs where it can be infused with more oxygen.

Only if we have taken a breath in, though.

In between breathing in and out we have a little pause. During this pause, the CO_2 builds up. Those chemoreceptors in the brain detect this rise in CO_2 and send impulses telling us to contract our diaphragm and allow us to take another breath in.

Of course, all this is magically going on in the body without us being aware of it.

So, back to the blue bloaters. These folks have permanently low levels of oxygen because of lung damage. Since oxygen and CO_2 work in tandem, one goes up one goes down, the CO_2 in their blood is always too high – this is known as hypercapnia.

After a while, the body gets wise to this and realises that high CO_2 are not a reason to trigger another breath, so it begins to detect the low oxygen levels in the blood as a trigger to the next breath. That's why, if you have COPD and have high CO_2 levels, giving you a high dose of oxygen can be dangerous.

People with COPD should always have their blood oxygen and CO_2 levels tested before being given oxygen and it is essential that the levels prescribed are kept to.

From Dawn's story you'll know it doesn't always happen like this! Dawn will also tell you about her fabulous non-invasive ventilator - - her Trilogy. This helps her because she is a CO_2 retainer and the ventilator increases the depth and volume of her breathing allowing more air to pass in and, importantly, out of her lungs so that she can clear some of that excess of CO_2 via the bigger exhalation. It is also hugely helpful because of her low lung function.

What about Pink Puffers then? Well, these guys somehow manage to increase their breathing rate to allow for the lower oxygen levels caused by the disease. They breathe fast – and when ill with an infection – even faster. Our normal breathing rate is about 10 -12 breaths per minute. It's not uncommon to see people with COPD, especially in an acute crisis, breathing at rates of 30 – 40 breaths per minute. That's a lot of effort there, just to maintain that rate of breathing. But the advantage of that is that oxygen levels are kept up, generally, and CO_2 levels are not too high. Pink Puffers blow off the CO_2. For these guys, high levels of oxygen are safe and sometimes necessary!

EXACERBATIONS

D awn has never been hospitalized with COPD - that's amazing! But what about flare ups? Do you get worsening symptoms?

What is an exacerbation?

There are two types of exacerbations. One with a fever, warning of sickness. The other with no fever, brought on by panic or environmental conditions.

If you have a fever, call your doctor. Now.

I was working at the London Hospital, Whitechapel, UK; when I began to specialise in respiratory physiotherapy. Mainly I was working with patients who were acutely unwell. Perhaps they were the victim of poor recovery after surgery, or maybe someone admitted with pneumonia or asthma after having an attack. Generally, they were people with COPD. Usually these would be people with known COPD, we often saw people we knew well!

When someone with COPD gets a chest infection on top of their COPD, we generally call it an exacerbation, or sometimes a flare up. Often it is hard to know when you are having an exacerbation, patients ask me if they need to see the doctor or is it just a "bad day"? Here's one definition of an exacerbation that might help.

"An acute exacerbation of chronic obstructive pulmonary disease (COPD), is a sudden worsening of COPD symptoms including (shortness of breath, quantity and color of phlegm) that typically lasts for several days."

What causes exacerbations?

An exacerbation can be triggered by several things. This pie diagram shows how exacerbations can be bacterial or viral or both.

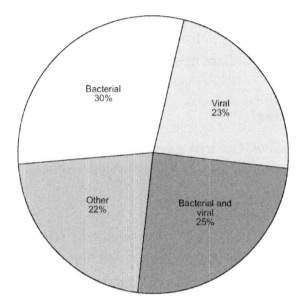

Papi A, Bellettato CM, Braccioni F, *et al.* Infections and airway inflammation in chronic obstructive pulmonary disease severe exacerbations. *Am J Respir Crit Care Med* 2006;**173**:1114–1121

Researchers think that exacerbations of bacterial and viral origin are often more severe and longer lasting than if only bacterial or viral.

The rest, or "other" may be a result of cold weather – cold bedrooms or outside temperatures may increase airway reactivity reducing lung volume. The British Lung Foundation suggests you aim to keep your bedroom temperature at around 18°C (64°F) and your living room at 21°C (70°F). These temperatures are warm enough to prevent viruses reproducing.

Air pollution can increase inflammation within the lungs so may also trigger a worsening of people's breathing. Antibiotics will be effective if there is a bacterial cause but not unfortunately if viral. Steroids and bronchodilators may help the symptoms in other exacerbations. Since over half of all exacerbations are likely to have a bacterial involvement in the UK we recommend that patients all have a rescue pack of corticosteroids and antibiotics so they can start treatment at the first signs. Don't you always seem to get worse over a weekend? Sometimes it's difficult to see a doctor quickly so if you have your rescue pack you can start treatment even before seeing the doctor.

If you have an exacerbation, one of the most important things you can do is to keep well hydrated. Mucus can get sticky fast! If your mucus is thick and sticky, steam inhalation can help – simply put a bowl of hot water on a flat surface and gently lower your face over it, and then inhale (so don't have the water too hot!) Maybe put a towel over your head to capture more steam. The steam then moistens your airways and loosens the sputum making it easier to cough up.

Some of us, ironically, cannot breathe in steam. An alternative is breathing through a warm, wet wash cloth. Breathe in, holding it over your nose. Take it away and gently blow. Repeat.

How do I know if I have an exacerbation?

Exacerbations can be defined by their symptoms, so if you know what to look out for it will help you manage them better – the earlier you get treated the better the outcome. Patients with COPD often have good and bad days and sometimes it is hard to tell if you need to start treatment. Monitoring your usual fluctuations in breathlessness, perhaps you are always worse when the weather is humid for instance, can help you know when to get additional help.

- Often people will complain of increased breathlessness doing their usual activities.

- You may cough more often than usual.

- You may notice a change in the color of your sputum (mucus) from clear to colored (deep yellow, green, or brown) and/or the amount of sputum that you bring up may increase. In many people, a change in sputum is the first sign that they have an exacerbation.

- There can be an increase in tiredness.

- A morning headache (that is unusual for you) can indicate that the blood CO_2 level may be a bit high and another sign of an exacerbation.

- If you regularly measure your oxygen levels, you may find they are lower than normal.

What does an exacerbation feel like?

I was seriously impressed with myself when I learned how to say the word "exacerbation".

I have learned that there are two types of exacerbations: those requiring a physician's attention, and those not involving a fever which we can often get under control ourselves.

If you have a fever, call a doctor. Immediately. As Rachel said, it is a wonderful thing if you have a doctor willing to give you a stash of Prednisone and antibiotics (we call the antibiotics a Z-pack). With a doctor's permission, you can begin treatment right away, rather than waiting until you can be seen and get prescriptions filled.

I now have a stash. As I was barely treated the first four years of my diagnoses, I went through pneumonia twice the hard way. The last time, by the time I made it to the doctor, I tried to sit in a chair in the waiting room and slid straight to the floor.

Pneumonia can take a COPD patient down quickly. It is crucial to begin treatment as early as possible. Any kind of infection needs addressed immediately with a physician. More on pneumonia later.

What is there is no fever? What if you flat-out cannot breathe? If there is ANY question of whether you can get this under control, call emergency services and get thee to a hospital.

Panic attacks can cause exacerbations. You panic, you cannot breathe, you cannot breathe, you panic. They feed off one another. People ask, "How do you know you are having an exacerbation?" You know.

I have asked people who have had exacerbations brought on by anxiety, bad air, or a combination of both, what happens at the hospital. They report that they are an anti-anxiety medication so that they can calm down enough to breathe. They are given a breathing treatment with an Albuterol nebulizer. They are usually kept overnight to ensure that they are stable.

My anxiety runs high – it is how my brain is wired. I take anti-anxiety medication. When I have an exacerbation not involving a temperature, I take my medication and sit on the floor with ice on the back of my neck. Cold makes it easier for many of us to breathe. I practice pursed lip breathing. Within a short time, I am breathing normally.

I believe that Klonopin has been a tool that has kept me out of the hospital.

If you believe that anxiety or panic effects your breathing, talk to your doctor about anti-anxiety medication. There are different types of anti-anxiety medication. Benzodiazepines are the most common. They can be addictive. If the inside of your head feels like a hamster on an exercise wheel, though, they normalize things. If I am having a panic attach and cannot breathe, I take a Klonopin, and calm down enough that I can use breathing techniques and breathe normally within a short time.

I feel nothing physically when I take Klonopin. The exercise wheel quits squeaking inside my mind. Some people, though, like the way they feel. Often, they like it too much. Unfortunately, this second type of person cannot take benzodiazepines without risking trouble with addiction. This is something you want to be honest with your doctor and yourself about.

There are also short-term sedatives that are not habit-forming.

This is NOT something to test out during an acute exacerbation. Call emergency services BEFORE you try to quiet an exacerbation with breathing techniques and/or medication for the first time. If your breathing is under control when they reach you, great. If not, get in the ambulance.

Medication can be abused. Self-honesty is as crucial, in its' own way, as an effective breath. I have struggled with addiction, and I have struggled with COPD. Even when I was one door away from death, COPD was easier. If you cannot take them as prescribed, leave them alone.

Most of us have Albuterol and nebulizers. The steam from the nebulizer will open your airways, making it easier to breathe. The Albuterol will do its' work.

Keeping your breathing under control with pursed lip breathing will help prevent an exacerbation of the second type. If you are out in the world and find it difficult to breathe, stop and lean on something. Smell a flower, flicker a candle. If someone asks if you are okay, do not waste your breath answering. Give them a thumbs up if you are okay. If you are not okay, ask them to call emergency services.

WHY DID I NOT KNOW THIS?

*T*he first part of pulmonary rehabilitation was education. This is where I found the answers to the questions I had relentlessly asked at the PMA.

I should have gotten it, after my first few appointments, that I may as well have stayed home and asked questions of a magic eight ball. "Reply hazy, try again".

Looking back now I was clearly on hospice. "Comfort care", which had little to do with comfort, and less with care. Without my knowledge, without my permission.

Four years into my diagnosis I saw a new doctor and things changed. Hospice must have dropped from my chart. I am now treated as a human being worthy of health care.

When I first hit rehab, though, I was thoroughly confused. Weak, and sick, and confused.

Alicia, Kristin, and Elizabeth were passionate in their work, which appeared to be us.

They answered questions. They answered not only the questions I asked, but they also answered questions that I had not though to ask. They shared information. They helped us navigate the does and don'ts associated with COPD. They managed to convey the fact that I could do something to not only live with my condition but to improve it. They laughed.

They engaged.

Every time I showed up at rehab, I felt like I was walking into a party. It was truly something to be celebrated – health professionals who were not trying to convince me that I was dead and did not have the sense to lay down.

I tell people on my COPD site that if they have access to a respiratory therapist, they have struck gold.

I also tell them that if rehab could bring me back from the dead, rehab could turn them into Spiderman (gender politics aside).

After few weeks, the education part ended, and the dreaded exercise part began. Except that by now, I was not dreading it. Those three women had managed to turn dread into a cautious excitement.

The weights were candy-coloured and fit nicely in my hands. They even had tiny one-pound weights. I went with something a little heavier, but not by much.

I was a bit leery. The "going down like a redwood tree" thing.

We exercise by chairs. ALWAYS have a chair with you when you exercise.

They told us that if the exercises became difficult, we could sit down. That was comforting.

The first time we exercised I wanted to sit down. I did not, because the eighty-nine-year-old woman next to me kept going.

We did an exercise. I did not keel over. We did another exercise. I glanced at Bethany, the elderly woman next to me. Any signs of slowing down? Nope.

Music played, people laughed. Elizabeth explained why we were doing the things we did. Some exercises open your airways, some strengthen your core muscles (which aid in breathing and weight loss), some strengthen your arms, your legs.

Simply put, the stronger your muscles are, the less oxygen they require.

*I kept thinking "I'll do one more", keeping an eye on Bethany. She **must** be getting tired. We got to the balance exercises, which did not require much energy. Then stretching, which just plain felt good.*

Then – we were done. Bethany never did wear down.

Bethany and I worked out together for a year. After we exercised, we got on the NuSteps and started our "What are you reading?" conversations.

*

A couple of times Bethany did not show up. When I saw her afterwards, she told me "I really feel it when I miss a day. I can't do that."

When a week went by with no Bethany, and she did not answer her phone, I worried. I have no idea why an 89-year-old Mormon woman was the one I bonded with, but I loved Bethany.

Tasha also loved Bethany. When we hit the two-week mark without seeing Bethany, Tasha circled the chair Bethany worked out at, lowered her head, and gave me a hard stare.

I said "Okay. I'll find her."

I found her at an assisted living, not being cared for. She had a stroke. When we walked into her room, Tasha walked up to the bed and touched Bethany's hand with her nose. Bethany stroked Tasha's head and cried.

Bethany signed some papers, which allowed me to throw a fit and make them care for her. I would walk down the hall and hear the staff whisper "It's the lady with the dog."

*

Groups are great. You have the "We are all in this together" vibe going on. Rehab with a group feels a lot like a party. We get to watch each other beat back this disease. We laugh. A lot.

They were not "show off at the gym" type exercises. They were small, targeted exercises designed to tone every part of our bodies. Balance exercises because we cannot fall. You have no idea how unbalanced you are until you do a balance exercise. The chair comes in especially handy on the balance exercises. You put your hand on the back of the chair, get in position, and lift your hand off the chair. It was quite some time before I was not grabbing the back of the chair every couple of seconds.

This is where Elizabeth shines, the exercise physiologist. She has a fantastic rhythm to her exercises. It was easy to fall into that rhythm, to stretch, warm up, strengthen. My body craved movement. The more I moved, the more I wanted to move. Exercise became a dance.

They took measurements when we started rehab. After six weeks of exercise, they took the measurements again and told us how much we had improved.

I did not need to be told.

I had been in the process of dying. The women at rehab literally gave me life.

I was practicing something at physical therapy one day and my PT told me "Stop that. You are mindfully exercising, not flipping your body about."

I said, "Oh. I have always just flipped my body about."

I applied that to the exercises at rehab. Simply paying attention to the muscles I was moving made the exercises more effective.

If you do not have a group, you will have to be a bit more disciplined. We are writing this book during the Covid pandemic. When the world closed, I got lazy for a week and did not exercise. I felt like I was going to die. Literally. I felt like my illness had moved into a deeper stage. I was exhausted, frustrated, and everything hurt.

One night I was lying in bed and realized that tears were rolling down my face. I had no idea how long that had been happening. I have a herniated disc *in my neck, and the stretches I did at rehab relieved pain in my neck and shoulders.*

I got up and grabbed my weights. Ten minutes into our rehab routine, the exhaustion and frustration lifted. It took a month to get the pain under control.

You can buy weights on Amazon, or you can use cans of soup. You do not even have to use weights if you dot want to. I use four-pound weights.

I do not do our whole routine every day, but I do a few exercises. I get my cardio at the dog park. Dogs have not been cancelled. We practice social distancing, the people. We stay at least three German Shepherds away from each other. I walk the track with my four magnificent beasts.

The dog park is also their rehab. These broken old dogs come to me, they hit the dog park and begin to age backwards. Tasha spent her first nine years in a cage as a breeder. She was nearly crippled when she first came here. I realized how much her health had improved when I was gathering leashes at the dog park and wondered why she was not frantically pushing to get out of the car. I looked up and she was running around in front of the car. She had sailed through the open window.

We walk the track at the dog park to keep them out of trouble. Many dogs that stand around get stressed and act out. With four dogs and 24% lung function I cannot afford to have one acting out. We walk, they run off and play for a minute and come back. If one of them tries to pull anything, they get a short time-out on a leash.

The Sheriff is fifteen-years-old and neutered. Despite this, he will once in a blue moon try to mount someone. I put him on a leash for a minute. He could care less. He stands there and grins like "Yeah – I still got it. I'm a bad dog on a leash."

The Sheriff is fifteen and acts like a three-year-old, because he works out at the dog park.

I am not allowed on the treadmill. My breathing changes, and Tasha will not have it. She pulls on my clothes until I get off the evil machine that is making me breathe funny. She is good with the Nu-Step.

Occasionally Tash checks out someone else, turns around and lowers her head, stares at me. Hard. I say, "You may want to check your saturation – my dog is looking at you funny." They do, and it is low.

Whoever is working with us walks around and checks in with us while we are on the machines. They check our saturation and heart rate, talk to us about whatever is going on. We do not have Kristin any longer, but she used to take an extra step. Almost absently, she would reach down and check the tanks of those of us who were using oxygen, to make sure we were not on the verge of running out. It touched me, that she thought of such things. I felt as though we were cared for.

I am looking forward to the world opening. They have allowed us back on the machines, but there is not enough room to work out and practice social distancing. I have not gotten a joke from Dave in a long time.

Reading through what Rachel has written, I understand a bit more about why all this works.

Toned muscles require less oxygen. A heart strengthened by cardio requires less oxygen.

Because of the pandemic, people have been locked in their homes, not moving around. It is getting hot. I do not know why, but it is hard to breathe when it is hot. I am seeing healthy people at the dog park struggle more than I do, with 24% lung function. Some of them are breathless, making it from their cars to the chairs in the park. I have limits and I must pace myself, but rehab literally brought me back from the dead.

I was in the process of dying when Patrick talked me into going to rehab. Every time I exercised it got a bit easier to exercise. Before I knew it I was walking the track at the dog park with my magnificent beasts.

(STAGES) SEVERITY

One thing to note here is about severity. Dawn has Stage 4, or even "end-stage" (horrible term) COPD but she thrives with COPD. I have seen folks with Stage 1 or 2, mild COPD, who struggle terribly with COPD. Stage is measured by lung function tests, and that is only one way of measuring COPD. Breathlessness can be bad with good lung function tests, or breathlessness may be manageable with terrible lung function tests. Symptoms such as anxiety can significantly impact an individual's ability to move and breathe (even if lung function tests are good). Rehabilitation can really help here too.

Back when I was frantically Googling, trying to figure out what was going on with my body and what I could do about it, I read about Stages.

All the internet explained is which lung function percentage was crammed into which Stage. To get your lung function they officially measure the amount of air you can force from your lungs in in a certain number of seconds.

*About that – the "blow-in-the-tube" tests. Many of us make ourselves miserable, trying to conjure of breath that is not there while someone yells "BLOW BLOW BLOW." During one such test, I ended up on the floor, retching, after the **fifth** time the tester repeated this. He then wanted me to get up and do it again. I left, falling several times before I made it back to the car.*

In the notes he left in my chart, he said I was "Uncooperative and antagonistic."

I lived in terror of those tests, until it occurred to me to tell them beforehand that when I am out of air, I am done blowing. No amount of yelling will conjure more air. The people who test me now are good with this.

Back when I was frantically Googling COPD to figure out what was going on with my body and if I had any control over it, the internet gave me dire information.

Do not Google.

This is standard on what the internet has to say regarding lung function under 30%:

*"Doctors call this "end-stage" **COPD**. That means you have very little lung function. Any new flare-ups could be life-threatening."*

I was diagnosed with 18% lung function. Things were not looking good for me. After a couple of years of rehab, I have improved to 24% lung function. The internet still says that I am in serious trouble.

I do not believe that "end-stage" is a thing, not until I have ordered a pizza and asked everyone to come say good-bye.

It means that nothing more can be done for a patient medically. I have found that there is always something more. The latest miracle is a portable non-invasive ventilator called the Trilogy, which I will be talking about later.

*(Then a **smaller** portable non-invasive ventilator called the Life2000. It just keeps getting better.)*

*Rehab completely turned my life around with exercise. I have figured out how to function within my limits and do not feel like I am missing out on anything. I covered just about **everything** in my life before COPD.*

I was basically on my own medically for a few years, other than my Facebook doctors. In some ways, that may have been a good thing. I needed to figure things out. When someone told me "That won't work" I did not listen, because I had become extremely tired of doctors trying to get me to hold still so they could shovel dirt on me.

When someone on the COPD page presented a clue, I dove in. I found out what worked and what did not. At times I got it wrong. When I started getting oxygen through a nasal cannula, I got congested and could not breathe through my nose. This is because oxygen dries out your sinuses and they swell – I did not know that.

The first couple of fixes I found turned out to be the wrong ones. I have spent many Friday nights studying mucus, and finally saw an excellent nurse practitioner.

I can breathe at night now.

Because my doctors for the first few years, and the internet, were insisting that I could keel over at any moment, I did not have the luxury of thinking that sinus rinses were too weird to try.

Because of this, I can breathe.

I do not have the luxury of simply not exercising when I do not feel like exercising. I did stop exercising for a week when the world closed for the pandemic. I felt like I was going to die. It was not the melodramatic "I'm gonna die!" I felt like my body was giving out on me.

I immediately got up and went through our entire routine. Exercise brought me back to life. Again.

NIV (NON-INVASIVE VENTILATION – A PORTABLE BREATH)

I just put on my Trilogy.

I can breathe.

All night this amazing thing will breathe for me. Deep, satisfying breath that fills my lungs.

I put it on as soon as my beasts and I have migrated to the bedroom. I write. I draw. I enjoy breathing.

That first deep breath was the most exciting thing that has ever happened to me.

I cannot describe how huge it is, not going to sleep every night wondering if this will be the night I stop breathing.

They are still relatively new to pulmonary medicine. Respiratory therapists know about them, but respiratory therapists know about everything. My old pulmonologist had no idea I needed one. Someone in my Facebook group prescribed one for me.

I was discovering that the sleepy and confused thing I struggle with was "CO_2 poisoning". High CO_2 levels. Having my oxygen turned all the way up that first couple of years did me no favors.

The pulmonologist I was seeing was a kind man. He had knowledge, but he had no interest in CO_2, though. He told me that if I had CO_2 issues I would not be able to hold my hand steady, at a right angle to my arm. It would flap.

I talked to him once about a friend who had sleep apnea and could not wear the CPAP mask. He had great ideas for other people. Me, he gave me inhaler samples and shrugged.

*How could I **still** be alive with no lungs?*

I told Facebook about the flapping hand thing. One of my premier Facebook doctors said, "He may be a nice guy, but you need to give him the flapping finger and get another doctor."

You cannot change doctors in my system. I tried. I did not want to leave the system and lose my rehab people.

The city I live in, Sacramento, is a bowl. When Northern California was on fire, we received all their smoke. I became so sleepy I was almost narcoleptic. I left several messages for my doctor. None were returned.

After a few weeks I tried making an appointment with another doctor. The other doctor's assistant looked at the computer and said, "But you have an appointment in a couple of months with your doctor."

I told her I was having problems now and could not get in touch with him. She called my doctor's assistant, who called me and made an appointment.

He put me on a course of Prednisone, a wonderful/awful drug that woke me up a little.

By now Facebook had told me about CO_2 and what I needed to do to deal with it. That is how it worked. Facebook diagnosed me, then I would try to get a doctor to do something about it.

I had told my Facebook group about the flapping hand thing. Patrick said, "You need to give the doctor the flapping finger and get another doctor."

You do not just switch doctors in my system, and I liked my doctor. He cared. He was willing to take a chance on me and give me a referral to pulmonary rehab, even though he did not think I would live long enough to make it through the wait list.

I asked my doctor to order an ABG, an Arterial Blood Gas, to find out where my CO_2 levels were at.

He looked at my hand.

I said "I know. My hand is not flapping. Everyone tells me that I need numbers, though."

He shrugged, willing to humor me.

On the way out, during the check-out process, I had to have someone run back and remind him to order the ABG.

(I recently got a look at my records. They are wildly inaccurate, but that is another thing. My doctor had written "Patient's primary care physician has told her that she needs an ABG."

Hopefully, Patrick is getting a laugh out of that, somewhere. He liked to laugh, to make us laugh.

We lost Patrick to something not related to COPD.)

That is the only time I have entered a hospital for something COPD related, was to have that blood draw. The internet tells me that COPD patients with under 30% lung function have been hospitalized at least once, and their next flare-up will probably be lethal.

I am not even close to 30%. Before rehab, I was 18%. After a couple of years in rehab, 24%. I have never been hospitalized, because of rehab. I know how to take care of myself, and I take the magic pill that beats back this illness. Exercise.

I brought my laptop with me, I had heard that ABGs were painful, and I thought I would distract myself by drawing on the computer. They needed one wrist to draw blood from, but I can draw one handed.

The woman drawing the blood said, "Big pinch."

I started thinking "That's not so ba…..Holy Cr*p!"

Yes, it hurt. It was done quickly, though. Everyone in the room (except for the one woman who was terrified of Tasha, snoozing on the floor) became interested in the dog I was drawing. I gave them a tutorial for a while, then realized I had been there almost an hour.

I asked "Are we done? Can I leave?"

Someone told me "We are waiting for your doctor to call. We can't let you leave. Your CO_2 levels are high."

The "can't let me leave" frightened me for a minute, but there was no way they could force me to remain in the hospital. I had grown weak that first couple of years, but exercise had brought my strength back. I was confident that I could break out if I had to.

I busted up laughing. I said "He's not going to call. To get ahold of him, you must call another doctor's assistant, then get them to call his assistant, then wait until he comes back in. He is getting ready to retire. He doesn't spend a lot of time in the office."

They let me go, although they were reluctant to part with the process of the dog appearing on my computer. Except for the woman who was terrified of my snoozing German Shepherd. Me leaving meant she could come out of hiding.

I somehow managed to get ahold of the numbers, and asked Facebook to interpret them.

Yes indeed, I had CO_2 poisoning. There is a fix for people who retain CO_2, which is a potential danger when you are on supplemental oxygen.

The Trilogy. A miracle of a machine. A non-invasive portable ventilator. You stick your oxygen tube on it. It measures the blood gases in your exhale and gives you the exact amount of oxygen your body needs. No more, no less.

Teri, one of my Facebook doctors, said "I prescribe the Trilogy with the DreamWear."

Ironically, The DreamWear headgear is what my doctor had pulled up on his computer for my friend with sleep apnea.

I asked him why my friend's doctors did not know about the DreamWear.

He chuckled. He said "They come out with new things all the time. You have to be kind of OCD about it."

I wondered why he could not be OCD about CO_2.

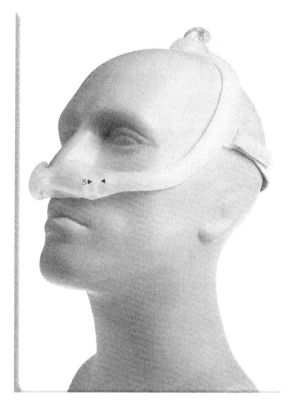

I had a diagnosis. I had a prescription for the fix. The problem: The Trilogy is a $10,000 machine. I had not been worth a 69-cent humidifier at that PMA.

My doctor was on the verge of retiring. My wonderful women at rehab had aimed me at a good doctor at a different PMA in the same system. I was not scheduled to see him for six months, though.

I met with my doctor one more time. I laid everything out and he tried hard to get me scheduled sooner with the new doctor. An appointment was made for a date a couple of weeks away.

I told my doctor I hoped that he spent a long time doing absolutely nothing. His career had impacted the world. He designed the pulmonary rehabilitation program that brought me back from the dead.

The new doctor's office called me and told me they were moving the date of the appointment back because I had just seen a doctor.

I said "The reason I saw him was to get the appointment with the new doctor moved up. I have CO_2 issues."

He asked, "What happened at the appointment?"

"The doctor ran from one computer to another and managed to get the appointment with the new doctor moved up."

"What did you discuss?"

"Getting the appointment with the new doctor moved up."

There was no moving the appointment up. I had to wait.

The new PMA was right upstairs from rehab. The rehab professionals were not allowed to give medical advice, but they managed to aim me at a good doctor.

At the old PMA, when I walked in, I stood at the reception counter for a while. Eventually the receptionist would glance at me, sigh, and go back to what she was doing. After spending a good deal of time shuffling papers, she would say "Date of birth."

They were not happy to see me. I do not know if it was because I insisted on living, or if they were not happy to see anyone.

The woman who took my vitals when I was finally admitted through The Door was great. My doctor's assistant had moments of greatness. My doctor was a kind man, and willing to humor me when I insisted on doing things that would keep me alive. There was one nurse practitioner who listened to me, once. It was after I had figured everything out through Facebook and rehab. If I had hit him in those first couple of years, I would not have suffered through the things I suffered.

Everyone else at that PMA, though – condescending was the best I could hope for. At my last appointment there with a nurse practitioner, I started mentioning something about rehab. I had been in rehab almost two years. He interrupted me and said, "You do NOT have the lung function to benefit from pulmonary rehabilitation."

I said, "I'm glad the people at rehab don't see it that way."

When I walked through the door at the new PMA, the woman at the receptionist greeted me as if I was an old friend. Her face lit up and she looked genuinely happy to see me.

I turned around to see who she was talking to. There was no one behind me. She was talking to me.

I was stunned.

I continued to be stunned. Every single person in that office treated me as a human being worthy of healthcare.

When they did the "blow in the tube" (spirometry) test, I told the woman doing the testing that when I was out of air, I was done blowing.

She smiled at me and told me that was fine.

The spirometer tests your lung function. My lung function had improved to 24%. That is not supposed to happen. My Facebook friend Ted pointed out that my lung function had increased by THIRTY PERCENT.

My new doctor treated me with respect. I told him about the CO_2 and gave him Teri's prescription. This was the defining moment.

He told me he would write an order for a Trilogy.

I had mentioned that my oxygen company had tried to kill me, and he went with another oxygen company.

Sel tells me "They did not try to kill you." I say, "Yes they did."

The next day I had a $10,000 machine sitting on my nightstand.

*They wanted me to wear a mask. I tried, for a while. When I put that mask on, the tech turned the machine on. My eyes got huge. I had **forgotten** what a deep breath felt like.*

He said "Oh! Is that too much?" and immediately turned the pressure down. It is hard to talk with a mask on, I kept trying to tell him "No! Turn it back up!" I finally took the mask off and said "No! Turn it back up!"

I could not wear the mask, for several reasons. The second I put it on I irrationally felt water deprived. I was water deprived for a while when I was a teen. In my car I have an open soda, a water bottle, a back-up case of soda in the back, water for the dog, and a back-up gallon of drinking water. I am not comfortable unless I have at least one thing to drink available. I often have three things going on at once. Water, coffee, and Ginger Ale.

My dog Burt was also water deprived, held as evidence in a cruelty and neglect case in which he was the victim. They kept him in a back room at a shelter for over a month, alone, covered in garbage, apparently without water for much of the time.

The first night he was here he tried to climb into the toilet, all 96 pounds of him. I said "No, Burt, we don't stand in the toilet."

He backed out of the toilet. He looked at me like "We don't? Okay." Looked back at the toilet, back at me. "It would be better if we did."

For two weeks, every time he drank, he put his foot in the water bowl to keep it from escaping.

I keep a bowl of water in the bedroom now. Before I did, Burt paced all night. He knew he could have water if he wanted to go get a drink, but he was not comfortable unless he could see a water bowl.

Like mother like dog. I get it, Dude.

If I did manage to fall asleep, I would wake up on the floor, convinced someone was trying to smother me. Another legacy from my teens. I have had an odd life.

I ordered the DreamWear headgear from Amazon. I did not know that Sleepcare Source would just bring me one. They have been amazing. Their service is almost instantaneous.

When a Trilogy RT was assigned to me, I spoke to her on the phone about the mask. She has a deep voice and a gender-neutral name, so I thought she was a man until I met her. She told me on the phone that only the full-face mask was effective.

I thought "One more man who has decided that he knows everything and there is no telling him different."

She came out to the house. I told her that the mask would not be effective if I could not wear it. Then I told her why. What was behind the struggling for my life on the floor as I woke up ripping the mask off.

When people talk about PTSD I often cringe. It has become a catch-all for many things that have nothing to do with true PTSD. I did not know if it truly applied to my situation and what I went through when I was a kid on the streets.

I had to tell her so that she would understand what happened when I put that mask on. It was not just claustrophobia. To my horror, I cried.

She said "Okay. I am fitting you with the DreamWear."

It is effective. I need a chin strap to keep my mouth closed when I sleep. If I open my mouth, I turn into a wind tunnel. It is amusing, but not effective. Occasionally I relax enough before falling asleep that bubbles pop out of my mouth. Some people might not be bothered by this. I feel like a goldfish. I slap a piece of medical tape over my mouth that peels off easily and painlessly.

The benefits hit immediately. The morning after the first night I slept with the Trilogy, I woke up, and stayed awake. For years, twenty minutes after I got up, I was so tired that I wanted to sit on the floor and cry. I did not, but I wanted to.

The DreamWear is extremely comfortable. I can talk, I can drink, I can wrestle with the dogs, I can live my life. Although I do feel like Snorkledorf with the tube coming out of the top of my head.

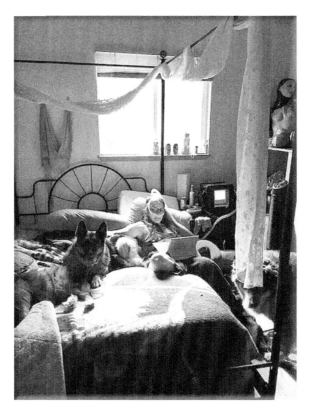

I had no idea that they not only dealt with CO_2, but greatly benefitted those of us with low lung function. I have been trying to figure out why. I have been reading medical studies. Most of them have been done in a hospital setting. As I said, Trilogies are new on the scene, and are not greatly understood in the field of pulmonary medicine.

This is a typical finding in a Trilogy study: **The addition of long-term NPPV to standard treatment improves survival of patients with hypercapnic, stable COPD when NPPV is targeted to greatly reduce hypercapnia.**

*In English, that means patients **survive longer** and are **less breathless**.*

That is huge. A COPD diagnosis is equated with increased breathlessness until the patient dies.

This is yet one more reason why "end-stage" is not a thing.

I slept without the Trilogy one night when I was congested. The next day I felt like I had a hang-over. I realized I always used to feel that way, pre-Trilogy.

I did not realize how much I struggle to breathe until just the other day, when I was talking to one of my wonderful rehab professionals.

When things are difficult, I tend to close my eyes and just do them. I shut down the part of my mind that says, "This is hard." It is a survival technique. Often not a survival technique that serves me well. After I have closed my eyes and barreled through something, someone will point out that there was an easier way to go about it.

For several years I worked three jobs. I worked seven days a week, sometimes eighteen hours a day. I gave camel rides at the zoo, tended to the animals at Fairytale Town, and waited tables at night. After one job I would take a quick shower and a nap and go to the next job. I did not think about how tired I was.

I was waiting tables one night and realized the family I was serving I had given camel rides to earlier in the day. The woman asked me "Are you everywhere?" I nodded. Yes, I was everywhere.

I talked to Elizabeth at rehab last week and asked her if she had any idea why I had so much more energy and it was so much easier to breathe even when I was not using the machine.

She talked about "the work of breathing". Pre-Trilogy, all night I struggled for breath. We breathe shallow when we sleep. My heart struggled to beat without enough oxygen. My brain struggled to heal without enough oxygen.

The Trilogy removed the work of breathing. I have near perfect lung function when I am on that machine.

Peewee always wakes me up ten minutes before the alarm goes off. Breakfast cannot be one minute late. I pull the covers over my head and enjoy filling my lungs for a few moments. Then I sit up and take the Trilogy off and put my oxygen tube on. When this happens, Burt goes into celebration mode. "It happened again! I'm still here! BEST DAY EVER!" Tasha usually gets off the bed while Peewee is urgently lobbying for breakfast. She gets back on the bed. It is not safe when Burt is celebrating.

When Elizabeth explained about the work of breathing, I realized how incredibly hard it is for me to breathe. It has become so much easier with my magic machine, but it is still hard. I have less than one quarter of a normal breath. Imagine putting a straw in your mouth, clamping your nose shut, and breathing through that straw.

I had been closing my eyes and ignoring that for a long time.

The machine is small, has a strap, and works off batteries for four hours. I have taken to bringing it into the living room.

Why struggle for breath when I do not have to?

Pulmonologists who have not kept up on research do not understand the benefits of the Trilogy.

A friend who has roughly the same lung function I do asked her doctor for a Trilogy. Her doctor refused. He told her "They discouraged patients from breathing on their own."

Seriously? We are too lazy to breathe?

The reverse holds true. The more you use the Trilogy, the easier it is to breathe when you are not using it.

Non-Invasive Positive Pressure ventilation (NIPPV) is an incredible device for people with COPD.

We kept people out of intensive care with it.

Patients would come into hospital struggling to breathe – increased work of breathing – and with high CO_2 levels in their blood (hypercapnia.) When you have COPD an infection on top can tip you over the edge. The work of breathing becomes so hard you simply cannot get a deep enough breath in to clear the CO_2 that builds up because of our natural metabolism. If CO_2 is high, oxygen will be low.

They work in tandem. Breathing becomes harder and harder until it is just too much.

The use of non-invasive ventilation (without the need for a tube down the throat) was first described in 1947. In World War II they used a device we called "The Bird"- because it looked a bit like a stork! This was termed Intermittent Positive Pressure breathing – the patient triggered the breath and "The Bird" added extra lung volume.

This device could not be strapped on. (I did try a makeshift strap once, but it kept falling off the patient's face!)

(This is why I love rehab professionals. I am picturing a determined Rachel Garrod with a willing patient and a couple of bungee cords.)

The machines we now know of as NIPPV did not become regular treatment until late 1980s.

When a person becomes hypercapnic their blood becomes more acidic. This change in pH. interferes with all the systems in the body.

It is essential to clear that excess CO_2.

NIPPV allows a deeper breath, triggered by the patient but completed by the machine. Some machines, like the Trilogy, also have a PEEP feature – the application of positive pressure at the end of an exhalation. This helps hold the airways open a little bit after the breath out (increased airway patency) making the next breath in easier.

Deeper breathing and easier inhalation ultimately reduce the work of breathing and resets the pH. blood level, giving the body the much-needed space to recover.

For some people, like Dawn, with long term hypercapnia (chronic high CO_2) sleeping with the machine means the deeper breathing overnight keeps her CO_2 at a regular level. The muscles involved in respiration are rested and not so easily fatigued, in turn making the next day a better breathing day.

In one of the studies I conducted, we gave one group of patients a NIPPV to use overnight and the other slept with oxygen. Both groups then took part in a pulmonary rehabilitation programme. The group that used the ventilators were able to exercise harder the next day and did better overall. We think that was probably because their breathing muscles were less prone to fatigue the next day.

If you have one and can use it during exercise it might help you do more. Speak to your doctor about it. If they prescribe one, it is worth persevering to get used to it and persevering to find the right mask.

Like Dawn says, "Why struggle for breath?"

Since I have written on this chapter, several changes have taken place in my life.

I lost The Sheriff, the alpha of the pack, who had been with me for sixteen years. Two weeks later I lost my beloved service dog Tasha.

The Sheriff earned his name at the dog park for breaking up dog fights. He would not have it when dogs went at each other. He was sniffing butts once and someone said, "Look! He's checking for priors!"

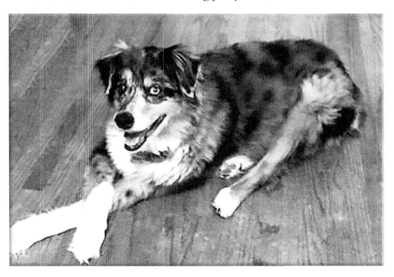

Mojo (The Sheriff) in his Mr. Casual pose.

I shut down emotionally for a while.

Chronic illness carries with it a unique form of depression. That worked in reverse with my diagnosis. I had been told I would be dead within days. I did not want to spend those days depressed, so I rewired my brain with cognitive therapy, by myself. I found myself freed from the fear and depression that had been life-long companions.

*I grieved Tasha in a way that I have never grieved anyone. I have never been as close to any other living being as I was with that dog. I let her in. She moved with me throughout my life, always. I sat on her dog bed for three months. I cried and watched all five seasons of **Downtown Abbey**.*

I finally realized that I had been sitting on my dead dog's bed for three months, and I got into therapy.

There is nothing wrong with asking for help.

Two days after I lost Tash, I lost Glenda. Glenda was like a sister, with all the convoluted trails of laughter and tears that meander through a sisterhood.

Glenda was here almost every day co-mothering the pack and making my life easier. She took The Sheriff on spa days, and snuck Peewee out and played with the water hose with her.

Peewee was a senior juvenile delinquent.

Tasha grew tired of watching me try to control Peewee at the dog park, so she put on her Police Dog hat and took over Peewee wrangling.

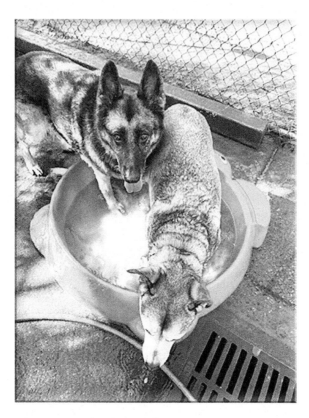

Tasha policing Peewee at the dog park.

Tasha did not approve of Peewee chasing after the hose. Tasha would snooze near me while Glenda snuck Peewee out back. Sooner or later there would be a telltale "yip" in the backyard, and Tasha would go and investigate.

I would hear Glenda say "Uh-oh, Peewee. Here come the cops."

Tasha would escort a wet, grinning Peewee back into the house.

We lost Peewee a bit over a month ago.

Dogs burn short, but oh, do they burn bright.

I have been taking in seniors and hospice dogs for six years. It is hard when they go, but it is such an honor to make their last days good ones. They have all given me more than I have given them.

They have never died all at once. The Sheriff, Tasha, Glenda, and Peewee. This has been beyond hard.

The house has been way too quiet. Peewee was a talker. That little face has been beside mine on the pillow every night for fourteen years.

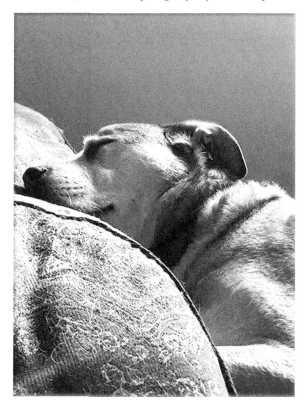

Again, I got depressed and quit exercising for a while.

Not okay. Not if I want to remain alive to be there for my remaining dogs.

When I picked up my weights, I realized again how much my body craves movement.

Burt has stepped up mas my unofficial emotional rescue dog, my knight in furry armor.

"I am just walking over to the coffee table Burt."

Burt is going with me to the coffee table.

"Okay. Put it in reverse. We are going back to the chair. You have got my tube wrapped around your nose. Yes, it is funny, but I need my tube. No, quit growling at your sister. It is not her fault that you have got yourself tangled up in my tube."

Dogs know.

I rescue them, then they devote every fiber of their being to rescuing me back.

My friend Matt said something once about feeling bad about laughing at Burt.

I said "Burt loves it when I laugh at him. He tries to figure out what is making me laugh, so he can keep doing it."

Matt said "Lawson, that dog has you spoiled rotten."

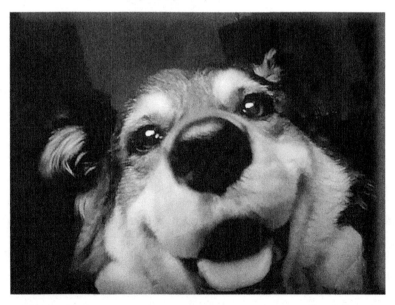

In the middle of all this something incredible happened.

I walked into rehab and set my weights on a chair. Alicia, our rehab coordinator, walked towards me with her eyes sparkling. She handed me a brochure.

That brochure changed my life. Again. End-stage? No.

My heart always broke a little when I got up in the morning and had to give up my Trilogy. I knew I had quite a few hours of barely breathing ahead of me before I could migrate back to the bedroom with the dogs and get back on the Trilogy.

Along comes the LIFE2000. A portable non-invasive ventilator. About the size that the first cell phones were. You wear it on a strap.

I have near-perfect lung function most of the time now.

My wonderful new doctor and his assistant worked with the rep from Hillrom, and she got this thing to me almost at the speed of light. She has been there with me every step of the way, the Hillrom rep.

The entire company has been with me every step of the way. Hillrom is something more than just a corporation. At least once a week someone calls to see how I am doing and ask if I need anything.

I had concerns about whether something so small could put out the volume of air the Trilogy gave me. This baby has volume.

When I get up in the morning now, I do not have to give up my breath.

We have come a long way from the day of the iron lung.

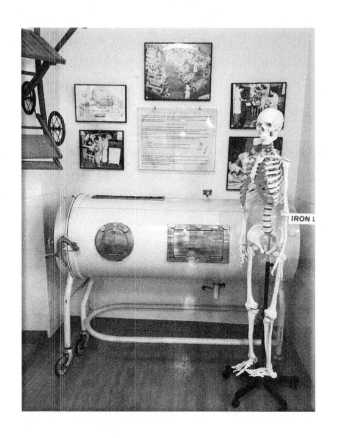

I did not look exactly like the guy in the picture when I was diagnosed, but close.

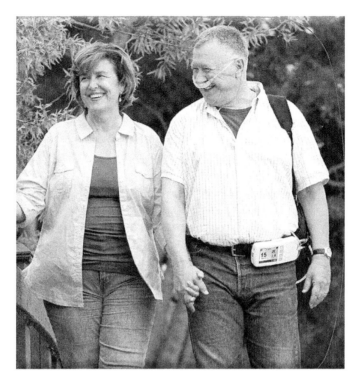

*There was a learning curve. But, hey, kindergarten was hard for the first few days. A breath is worth **everything**.*

The cannula is larger. It must be – it is literally giving you breath. I got used to that quicky.

The tube took me a few days to figure out.

I kept ¼" split braided cable around my oxygen tube to keep it from tangling and kinking. I tried that with the beefier Life2K tube. It made the tangling worse. I felt like I was participating in Sumo wrestling until I figured it out.

Being a writer, at the time I was thinking that the Tangling of the Tubes would make for a great short story.

They were giving me breath, but I was so tangled that I felt like the Michelin Man. (Google it.)

Instead of getting rid of the ¼" braided cable, I put ¾" split braided cable around the whole mess. I have no idea why I thought that would be a good idea. I felt like I was wrestling with an extremely long python.

Sel walked by once when I was utterly wrecked from tube-wresting. He asked me what was wrong. I said "Tubes."

Now it is all so easy that I cannot remember what the fuss was about.

I got rid of the cable that is so great for oxygen tubes.

I tweaked the design a bit. I tweak the design on pretty much everything but the dogs.

I wanted the device to swivel when I moved. I bought a cross-body strap from Amazon, and a swivel hook. I put a keychain ring on the zipper of the pouch, attached the swivel hook to the keychain, then clipped the swivel hook to both ends of the strap.

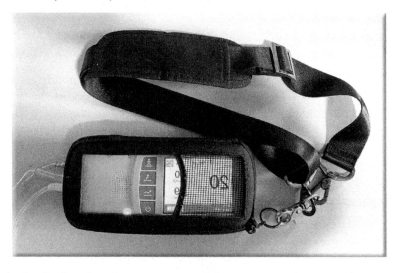

It swivels nicely when I move now and does not tangle as much.

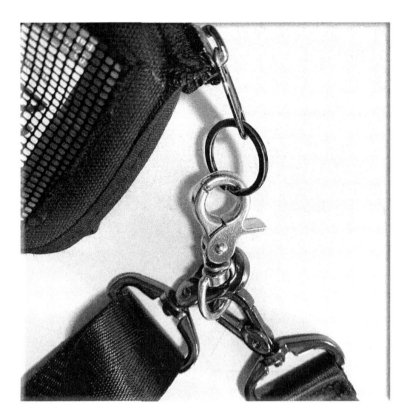

I have taken to wearing it around my hips, like an old-fashioned gunslinger wore a holster. It gives me a bit more mobility.

At the end of the day, I put on my portable oxygen for a few moments and untangle the tube.

Once you get the hang of it (literally – using gravity) it almost untangles itself. I remove one end of the tube from the little concentrator. I leave the other end attached to the device itself. Then I simply hold the tube up and run it through my fingers. The part that attaches to the concentrator weights the tube a bit, and the tube carries its' own weight, so it unwinds itself as I am running my fingers down the tube. I toss the unwound part over my shoulder to keep it from getting intertwined with the part that is unwinding.

Easy.

The tube coming from the cannula tangled for the first few days. I turned around in circles a few times unwinding it. You know what happens when you turn around in circles for any length of time.

I would try to land on a dog bed.

Without even being consciously aware of it, I learned how to move so that the cannula did not wind itself around me.

It has become as simple as walking around with an oxygen tube.

How miraculous, a deep breath. Sometimes I close my eyes and marvel at my lungs filling with air, over and over.

I used to have to force myself to exercise. I did not want to exercise until a few moments into my routine, when I realized, again, how much my body craves movement.

Breathing with the Life2000, I feel like exercising.

Migrating from the living room into the bedroom with my pack used to leave me exhausted. The computer needs moved, I need to lay in supplies to alleviate the PTSD Burt and I deal with from water deprivation, food needs to be heated up, one last round of drugs for dogs needs to be handed out.

Now I am breathing as I am doing those things – I get to the bedroom and I do not feel the need to collapse. I have the energy to write or draw.

***Everything** is easier when you can breathe. Who knew?*

There is no humidifier on the Life2000. My epic nurse practitioner Sossy Farajian gave it some thought and came up with an answer – a $15.00 personal humidifier from Amazon. It lives in a glass of distilled water on my bed stand.

If you have a Life2000, keep a hand towel over it so the mist cannot get to it. The water vs. electricity thing.

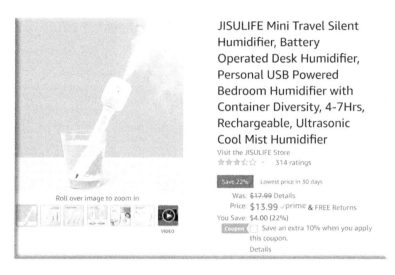

JISULIFE Mini Travel Silent Humidifier, Battery Operated Desk Humidifier, Personal USB Powered Bedroom Humidifier with Container Diversity, 4-7Hrs, Rechargeable, Ultrasonic Cool Mist Humidifier

Visit the JISULIFE Store

★★★½☆ ▾   314 ratings

Save 22%   Lowest price in 30 days

Was: $17.99 Details

Price: $13.99 ✓prime & FREE Returns

You Save: $4.00 (22%)

Coupon ☐ Save an extra 10% when you apply this coupon.
Details

Roll over image to zoom in

VIDEO

Personal Humidifier also in Tricks and Hacks

I fully acknowledge that my decision to pick up cigarettes when I was fourteen years old was a bad one. I understand the rage of that first diagnosing doctor. I do not like it, but I understand it.

I know people with COPD who still smoke and hate themselves for smoking. They are convinced they cannot quit. I understand that also and feel for them.

I "tried" quitting for decades. It turns out that the hardest part of quitting was making the decision to put them down for good. Once I finally made that decision it became so much easier.

What I had spent my life doing, in trying to quit, was to see how long I could go without a cigarette. I knew I would smoke again. I was convinced that I could not quit. Cigarettes were my best, sometimes my only, friend.

Alan Carr has a great book out about giving up smoking. He compares an addiction to cigarettes with a tapeworm. Every cigarette you smoke sets up the next craving, feeds the tapeworm. When you have made that decision, every craving you resist starves the tapeworm and makes the next craving weaker.

The "trying to quit" thing is a nightmare. That, and "cutting down". It leaves you laser-focused on the next cigarette. That overrides most everything else in your head.

I am grateful beyond words to the medical professionals in my life who do not believe that long-ago bad decision does not mean that I am unworthy of healthcare.

Of course, I would prefer the ability to fill my lungs on my own. I took away my lungs' ability to do that.

The Life2000 is utter magic for people such as me.

If your lung function is under 50%, or if you are a CO_2 retainer, you qualify for a Trilogy or a Life2000. You have the Trilogy in the UK. The Life2000 has not made it over there, but they are working on other portable non-invasive ventilators.

Many doctors do not understand them. A friend's pulmonologist told her he would not give her a Trilogy because he believed "They discouraged patients from breathing on their own."

Seriously? We are too lazy to breathe?

The opposite holds true. The more you use it, the better you breathe when you are not using it.

Find a rep from a Trilogy provider and ask your doctor to work with them. Or switch doctors if you can. Teaching hospitals care about current research and stay up on these things.

If you are in the United States and want to speak with someone about the Life2000, you can reach Hillrom at 1-800-426-4224. Dial 0. Talk to a rep, and ask your doctor if they would be willing to work with that rep. They have another extension for physicians.

Struggling for breath can be a thing of the past.

COPD Tricks and Hacks

From COPD Survivors around the Globe

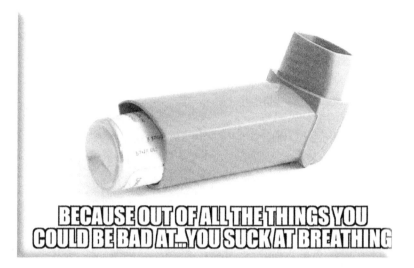

1) *Do you know how to breathe? "Pursed Lip Breathing" is the most effective way to take a breath. Your goal is to get oxygen in and CO_2 out. A good exhale is crucial for a good inhale. Breathe from your belly, not your chest. Take a deep breath through your nose, purse you lips, and GENTLY blow for twice as long as the inhale. "Smell a flower, flicker a candle flame." It is good practice and will help get your breathing under control during an exacerbation.*

2)   Pulmonary Rehabilitation will not only keep you alive, it will allow you to thrive. If rehab is not available to you, there are lots of YouTube videos under COPD Exercises. Move around. Safely. Faster does not mean better. DO NOT go fast for a mile, then not be able to get back home. Occasionally patients will be told that they do not have enough lung function to benefit from rehab. That is not true. Rehab took me from 18% lung function to 24% lung function, and literally brought me back from the dead.

3)   *The Portable Nebulizer is here! You will be more likely to use your Albuterol if you do not have to haul out a machine. Look at reviews on Amazon.*

4)   *Mucus and phlegm. If you suffer from stubborn mucus or phlegm, Mucinex or generic Mucus Relief will be your new best friend.* **100% Guaifenesin.** *You do* **not** *want "multi-symptom". They add speed to that, and it makes everything worse.*

Water is crucial if you take Mucus Relief tablets. Water is crucial if you are dealing with stubborn mucus or phlegm. Have I said "Water is crucial" enough to drive the point home that water is crucial?

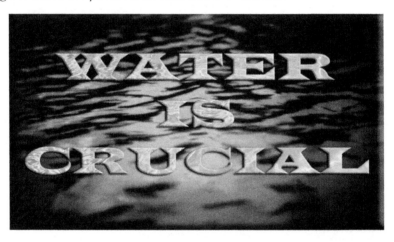

To get rid of lung phlegm, here is a link that explains devices. I call it the Flutter thingy. That is probably not the Latin term. https://www.youtube.com/watch?v=ZfanuH-SyPA

They also have compression vests. If you have a willing friend, you can ask them to cup their hands and **lightly** *run them up and down your back.*

The "Huff" method of coughing can be effective in bringing phlegm up. Lean forward and say "Hff!" as loud as you can. Huff without the "u".

5)   *For sinus mucus, sinus rinses can be a miracle. Sinus rinses sound weird, but they are great if you want to breathe. No, you will not drown.* **Distilled water only!**

There are several devices you can use. Doing contortions with the Netti Pot is no longer necessary. There is a $10 squeeze bottle. You push a button on the Sinugator, and it shoots water up one nostril and out the other. Prices vary. Walgreens has one for about $25.00. Walmart charges over $100 for the same thing.

They now have nasal irrigation systems that hold 16 ounces of distilled water and have 10 speeds. I settled on the SinuPulse. After I use it, I blow an extra 50 points on the Peak Flow. A breath will do you no good if there is nowhere for it to go. KEEP YOUR EQUIPMENT CLEAN. THIS IS CRUCIAL. I spray rubbing alcohol on the machine before and after I use it, and the spoon I use to mix the packets in.

5 ½)   *Nasal Rinse machines come with little packets of powder to mix into the distilled water. You can make your own. For every 8 oz of water, add ½ teaspoon of baking soda and ½ teaspoon of non-iridized salt.*

Cold water is unpleasant. For 8 oz, I nuke it for 30 seconds. For 16 oz, I nuke a coffee cup of distilled water for one minute, then mix room temp water out of the jug into the reservoir.

5 ¾)   *Apple Cider Vinegar. A friend mentioned on our site that he drinks Apple Cider Vinegar, and that he has no phlegm. This got my attention. You want the kind with "The Mother" ingredient, a chain of enzymes. It will say so on the bottle. I have spent years dealing with an avalanche of mucus. I started drinking Apple Cider Vinegar and took my tissue habit down from over a box a day to 2-3 boxes a week. Two teaspoons are recommended in a glass of warm water, with honey. It has proved effective for several people on our site. It has been in recorded use for over 2000 years, beginning with Hippocrates, the father of modern medicine. Marketers have*

gotten ahold of it and claim it can turn you into Spiderman. It cannot turn you into Spiderman. For some of us, it is hugely effective at getting rid of mucus and phlegm.

One of our members has reported that Apple Cider Vinegar works in pill form, also, if you cannot take the taste. I like the way it makes my sinuses spring open. It has been well documented that I am weird, though.

5 ½)   Apple Cider Vinegar also turns out to be great for your skin. It faded the prednisone spots on my arms and has kept them faded.

6)   Arm & Hammer has a great saline spray with eucalyptus, a natural decongestant. It is marketed as "nighttime", probably because that is when people are often congested. It is non-medicated. It breaks up mucus and keeps your nasal passages from drying out.

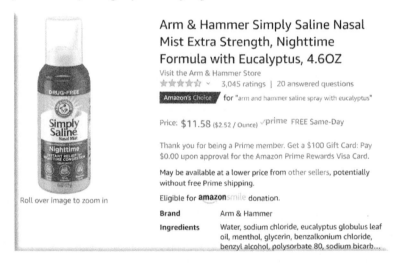

Arm & Hammer Simply Saline Nasal Mist Extra Strength, Nighttime Formula with Eucalyptus, 4.6OZ

Visit the Arm & Hammer Store

★★★★☆ ˅   3,045 ratings | 20 answered questions

Amazon's Choice for "arm and hammer saline spray with eucalyptus"

Price: **$11.58** ($2.52 / Ounce) ˅prime FREE Same-Day

Thank you for being a Prime member. Get a $100 Gift Card: Pay $0.00 upon approval for the Amazon Prime Rewards Visa Card.

May be available at a lower price from other sellers, potentially without free Prime shipping.

Eligible for amazon smile donation.

Brand	Arm & Hammer
Ingredients	Water, sodium chloride, eucalyptus globulus leaf oil, menthol, glycerin, benzalkonium chloride, benzyl alcohol, polysorbate 80, sodium bicarb...

Breathing through a warm, wet washcloth can also relieve congestion.

7)   To keep your tube from tangling and kinking, when you unwrap it, toss it in the drier on hot for one minute. Take it out and immediately unwind it. It will slither around nicely behind you. If you want a great tube that does not tangle and kink, Google "violet crush resistant low memory oxygen tube". Look at a few. The violet ones are all the same, but prices vary.

I keep the violet ones in the drier for 2 minutes, because they are thicker. Unwind it IMMEDIATELY, so it does not cool tangled. A lingerie drier bag for will keep the hose from tangling in the drier. I got 3 for under $8.00 on Amazon. You can also pick them up at a Dollar Store.

EDIT: They sell split braided cable, ¾ inch, on Amazon. I put it around my tube and tangling, kinking, and getting stuck on a blade of grass are a thing of the past. The tube will try to escape. I lightly wrap duct tape around it every few feet, and tape it to the tube at the beginning and the end. Start the cable down past your cannula, so you can switch out the cannula when it becomes brittle or take the cannula off and attach the tube to a machine if you use a machine. Make sure it is braided cable. The plastic ribbed cable makes a hideous noise as it follows you around.

8)   There is a chance everyone already knows this, but I did not know that a humidifier on your concentrator existed until two years into my diagnosis. That was two years of waking up every morning with a bloody pillow. Again, DISTILLED WATER ONLY. When your nasal passages dry out, they swell, and it is hard to breathe. If you need more moisture, there is an inexpensive gel called Ayr at most drug stores.

9)   Clean your humidifiers once a week with 50% white vinegar and 50% water. If you use a CPAP or Trilogy, clean the nose piece or mask daily with Dawn dishwashing soap.

*10)   Stay away from cleaning chemicals, **especially** bleach. Use white vinegar instead. If you need to kill germs, use rubbing alcohol.*

11)   Keep the air in your home clean. Invest in good filters for central heat and air. Put a small air cleaner where you spend most of your time. Do not open windows on bad air days or during storms. In the States most of us can check the air by punching AQI (air quality index) and your zip code into a search engine. No fires unless you have an insert that will not let smoke escape. Beeswax candles only, unscented. Paraffin candles release toxic chemicals as they burn. So can scent added to beeswax or soy candles. You can also get a candle wax melter and melt 100% soy wax. Make sure it is 100%. Soy wax burns cleanly. You can add vanilla extract and to room will smell fabulous.

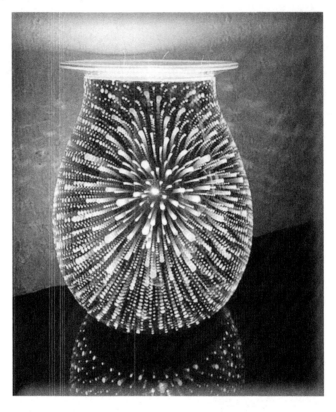

If you miss fires, they have inexpensive electric fireplaces out now.

12)   Non-essential organ. If you suddenly find yourself standing in a puddle of urine, your body has decided that your saturation is too low to keep everything going and has done away with your bladder. Most insurance, including Medi/Medi, will pay for products with a doctor's prescription. Bladder control products will arrive in a discreet box. Most pulmonary doctors are unaware that this is a common symptom of COPD. If this is happening to you and your pulmonologist does not know this is a symptom, please educate them.

Shethinx.com also sells absorbent, washable women's underwear.

13)   Pace yourself. Keep 2 pulse oximeters, one for home and one to keep with you. If your saturation drops, lean against something, or sit down. If people want to know if you are okay, do not waste your breath talking. Give them a thumbs up.

If you are unsteady on your feet, get a walking stick. I had a friend who used a walking staff decorated with feathers and beads and she looked like a high priestess. Rock your equipment.

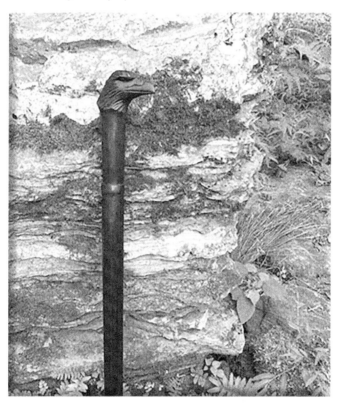

You can also get lightweight Aluminum Hiking Poles. The advantage of a staff, a walking stick, or a hiking pole is that you can stop and rest any time you want to, leaning on the pole.

*Any good doctor will tell you the secret to good health is **do not fall.***

14)   Try to stay out of hospitals, out of crowds, out of large gatherings of small children, otherwise known as germ machines. Getting sick can kill you. If you need to sit in an ER, carry an alcohol spritzer or hand sanitizer with at least 60% alcohol and disinfect your hands after touching anything the public has handled. Take a sheet with you to keep between you and whatever you are sitting on or leaning against. You may look paranoid, but you get to live.

Most pharmacies have hand sanitizer stationed every couple of feet, because they know. Use it. Again, you may look paranoid, but you will not catch whatever the last person handling that pen had. Be aware that many people cough in their sleeves. Then they want to hug you. Aim your little bottle of rubbing alcohol at them.

15)   After wearing a whole lot of cannulas that felt like plastic was eating my face, I found a great one, with small soft tubing that comes down over your cheeks. Google Westmed REF 0556.

There is also a company that makes an extremely soft cannula. https://www.softhose.com/

16)   Exercise to stay toned and limber and get your blood moving, but conserve energy where you can. Instead of wandering around shopping, most Walmart Groceries have a service now where you can order and pay on a computer and have everything delivered to your car the next day. Free, and the prices are good. Amazon is starting to offer this grocery service also. I get almost everything on Amazon. With prime, their prices are competitive.

17)   Instead of getting furious at your tube, make fun of it. If it will be funny later, it is funny now. Most things can be funny, even if they are painful. I have found that when I laugh at it I have it beat. Or you can be furious with your tube.

18)   Carry a back-up tank. Also keep an extra cannula in the car. I had one that got a hole poked in it and had no idea why my saturation was dropping like a stone.

If you use gas tanks, keep back-up O-rings. It was an O-ring that brought down the Challenger. If you put your oxygen interface on a new tank and oxygen hisses furiously out of it, that means that your O-ring has either worn down is laying on the floor somewhere.

19)   If your saturation keeps dropping and you cannot figure out why, put on a back-up tank and investigate. Check your hose to make sure it is not kinked. It may be time for a new hose. Check the air filter in the back of your concentrator. If it has been over 6 months, ask you 02 company to come out and clean it, or change it. Make sure the lid on your humidifier is on correctly. That tube also needs to be changed occasionally. I spent a week with my saturation plummeting and did all this. It turned to be the swivel connector between my cannula and my 50' hose. KEEP EXTRA CONNECTORS. Theoretically, swivel connectors help keep the tube from tangling. Sometimes they fall apart. They have a shelf-life. My 02 company said the shelf-life "should" be 6 months. Should-be-6-months, for me, turned out to be 2 months.

I like the rigid connectors. Not only do they not come apart, they hold the tubes together better.

20)   If you have dogs or busy little children, keep a death grip on your cannula to keep it from being yanked off your face. My 96-pound dog Burt considers it his sacred duty to follow directly behind me and stand on my tube.

21)   One of the common side-effects of Prednisone in bruised skin, and skin that splits if you look at it funny. Diabetic Lotion helps. Equate has a generic brand. Lately I have developed spots. Eczema crème helps fade the spots. (As well as Apple Cider Vinegar, applied externally.) Another

129

random side effect can be wanting to rip people's heads off or eat the refrigerator. Ask people around you to be patient with you.

22) If you use an inhaler containing a steroid, rinse your mouth AND gargle afterwards. You do not want thrush in your throat. This can result in a feeding tube. If you want to be thorough, rinse and gargle with warm salt water.

23) Optional. Find one thing you enjoy doing and do it. As often as you can. Then find another thing. If you like to travel and you cannot, consider getting an Oculus Go. You can meet up with your grandkids in Virtual Reality and be the cool grandparent, the one kids WANT to spend time with. You can also download a program called Wander, travel the world, and pick out spots to meet Facebook friends. I met my kid underwater in Hawaii the other day. We followed yellow fish around while we talked about how to be people.

24) It is not just you — showers are hard. Use a shower chair if you must. Keep a terry cloth robe outside the shower, and just put it on, rather than standing there drying yourself. Sit down for a bit if you need to. I wash my hair in the sink and take a million sponge baths. My roommate is threatening a washcloth intervention.

25) If you find yourself unusually sleepy or confused, talk to your doctor about the possibility that you are retaining CO_2. CO_2 levels can rise from too much oxygen, as well as too little.

26) If you are on Medicare and are having problems with your health care, Medicare has advocates. https://www.medicareadvocacy.org/

27) Singing along with the radio at the top of your lungs is a great way to exercise your lungs. Blowing up balloons and playing the harmonica are also good ways to exercise your lungs.

Singing does several things to benefit your health. It improves lung function. Singing releases endorphins, reducing pain. Studies have shown singing to boost your immune system. Those who sang showed higher levels of immunoglobulin A, an antibody your body secretes to help you fend off infections. Studies have also shown singing improves your mood. I do not need studies to tell me the last part – if I sing in the car long enough, I feel as though I have been through therapy. Singing also helps with grief, which I can attest to. Singing has been shown to improve memory in dementia patients.

28)   90% of a nasal spray's effectiveness lies in the TECHNIQUE in which it is used. Use a nasal spray with a Corticosteroid in it, like Flonase. Lean forward, spray it up towards the front of your nose. Do not sniff hard. Keep your head leaned forward for a minute, letting it sit there. I go so far as to rotate my head from side to side, and turn it upside down, so it can drain into my sinuses.

*29)   ***Do **not** use Afrin or Sudafed for more than 3 days. They work, for a minute, but they are heroin for the nose. You become addicted to them and they stop working, causing "rebound congestion".****

30)   Pineapple juice, or fresh pineapple, has proven five times as effective as most cough syrup. It contains the enzyme bromelain, which has anti-inflammatory properties. This usually does not get peoples' attention until I post a picture.

PINEAPPLE JUICE IS FIVE TIMES AS EFFECTIVE AS COMMERCIAL COUGH SYRUP.

It contains the enzyme bromelain, which has anti-inflammatory properties.

31)   The same meds that give you "dry mouth" (all of them) will also dry out and inflame your sinus passages. Stay hydrated! There is also a product for dry mouth called Biotene that comes in a spray or lozenges. Xylimelts are also a great product for dry mouth.

32)   If you need a "down day", take one. Some days, the best you can do is breathe in and out. That is okay.

33)   Sleep is crucial. For one, sleep debt looks exactly like severe anxiety to your brain. For another, during REM sleep the neurons in your brain flatten by 60% and spinal fluid rinses out molecular waste. I do not know what molecular waste building up in your brain looks like, but it cannot be good.   Here   is   the   article: https://www.nationalgeographic.com/magazine/2018/08/science-of-sleep/

34)   THIS is the important one. If you are a CO_2 retainer, or if you have low lung function, the Trilogy non-invasive ventilator is nothing less than a miracle. The hockey mask is not necessary. I use the DreamWear headgear. It has tubes that run down the side of your head and a little silicone piece that rests under your nose. The tube seeming to come out of the top of your head does look a bit funny. That first deep breath was the most exciting thing that has ever happened to me. It breathes deeply for you all night, and any other time you want to use it. Breathing is flat-out fun. If you use the DreamWear, you need a chin strap to keep your mouth closed. Otherwise, you turn into a wind tunnel. This can be amusing, but not effective.

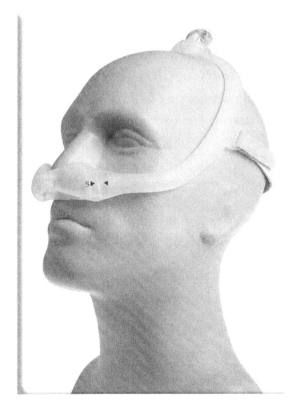

You can also use the DreamWear headgear with a BIPAP or CPAP machine if you have sleep apnea.

EDIT: In the States we have a great new device called the LIFE2000. A portable non-invasive ventilator. I wear it around my waist and have near-perfect lung function most of the time.

It has not made it into the UK yet, but there are different prototypes in the works. Check with your oxygen provider.

If you are a CO_2 retainer, or if you have under 50% lung function, you qualify for a Trilogy or Life2000. Medicare needs specific language on the script. Ask your doctor to work with a representative.

More about both devices in the NON-INVASIVE VENTLATION chapter.

35)   IF YOU STILL SMOKE: STOP! Stopping smoking (along with pulmonary rehabilitation) is THE MOST IMPORTANT treatment to prevent deterioration of your lungs. If you cannot do it alone (or it just feels too hard) get help. Patches help, as well as nasal sprays, gum, lozenges. There are medications available. Champix and Zyban, or you can try the herbal supplement CYTISINE (this is great, safe, and cheap -- get it from Amazon.) Group support helps. Facebook has many groups, or your doctor may be able to refer you.

36)   Balance is hugely important. Healthy people go down and break a hip and end up with pneumonia. We cannot afford to break things.

There are balance exercises in the exercise videos. You do not know how unbalanced you are until you do them.

If you need a walking stick, get one. If you need a walker, get one. Walkers nowadays can sport wheels, seats, and cup holders. If you need a scooter, get one. Scooters can be fun.

A group of us went to the California State Fair with a friend who had mobility issues. We all kept stealing her scooter and had a great time.

37)   **PLAN AHEAD**. *If you depend on an electric concentrator to live, a generator is not a luxury item. A small generator, enough to power your oxygen and a light, is a must.*

38)   *Sleeping position. The best position for you to sleep in if you have respiratory issues is on your side, with a pillow between your legs and your head elevated. If fluid is collecting in your lungs, as in pneumonia, sleep as upright as possible. Wedge pillows are great.*

39)   *Fear. A psychologist friend taught me a trick: fear and excitement generate the exact same chemical compounds in your brain. When you are scared, find something to aim excited at, and you will become excited. Terrified of what may come with your MRI results? You are excited about knowing exactly what is going on with your body and taking steps to deal with it. When Rachel is on a plane and dealing with turbulence, she pretends she is on a roller coaster. She is the passenger screaming "Wheee!" while everyone else is trying to figure out if their seats will indeed become flotation devices.*

40)   *HUM Breathing. Simply hum while you exhale. The American Journal of Respiratory and Critical Care Medicine have found that Nitric oxide, a beneficial gas produced in the sinuses, increased 15-fold during humming. Hum breathing reduces congestion and keeps the sinuses healthy. Aim for ten to twenty "hum" exhales.*

41)   *Find yourself allergic to your oxygen cannula? There are cannulas that do not touch your face on Amazon. Enter the words "Oxygen Diffuser Cannula."*

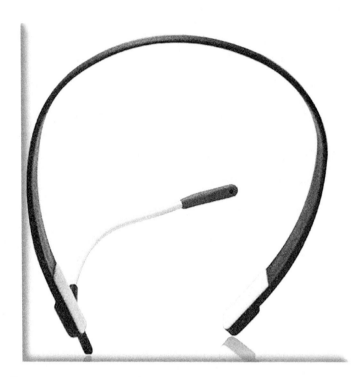

42)   *Do not put your underwear on over your tube. This never works out well.*

43)   *If you need a machine to help you breathe and cannot afford one, Google The Reggie White Foundation. They help people pay for machines.*

44)   *If you need help in general, whether it be paying your bills, mental health, finding a doctor, 211.org is a great resource.*

45)   *There is a Facebook page for those experiencing lingering COVID symptoms, Long Haulers.*

46)   *If you need help around the house Google your state and "In Home Support". They may have it, and you may qualify. In Home Support pays people to clean your house, help with errands, do things to keep you out of assisted living.*

47)   Occasionally your local Lyons Club will give you help if you need it.

48)   Acid reflux is the third leading cause of asthma. If you have acid reflux, treating your reflux will help your breathing.

49)   HEAT. Many of us find it hard to breathe in the heat. When I go to the dog park when it is hot, I keep an ice pack in my pocket. If I get overheated, I put the ice pack on the back of my neck.

When I am sitting down, I have an ice pack in a thin towel underneath one of my thighs. When I am laying down, one under my thigh, one behind my neck.

Neck fans are great. I wore one to the dog park and thought, "There is a nice breeze out." Oh yes – the neck fan.

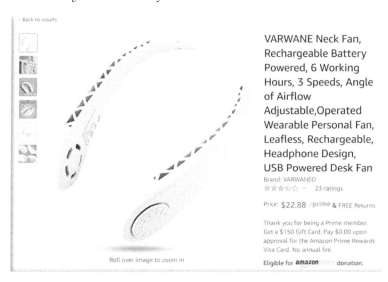

VARWANE Neck Fan, Rechargeable Battery Powered, 6 Working Hours, 3 Speeds, Angle of Airflow Adjustable,Operated Wearable Personal Fan, Leafless, Rechargeable, Headphone Design, USB Powered Desk Fan
Brand: VARWANEO
★★★☆☆ ˅   23 ratings

Price: $22.88 ✓prime & FREE Returns

Thank you for being a Prime member. Get a $150 Gift Card: Pay $0.00 upon approval for the Amazon Prime Rewards Visa Card. No annual fee.

Roll over image to zoom in   Eligible for **amazon** donation.

Personal humidifiers are like miniature swamp coolers. I purchased one for humidity at night for the Life2000. To my delight, it puts out a cool mist. Sel has one in front of his fan. **Distilled water.**

If you have a Life2000, keep a hand towel over it. The water vs. electricity thing.

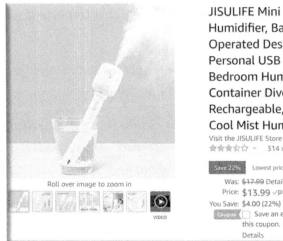

50)   *Changing the bed. As with the shower, changing the sheets is a thing for many of us. I do not know why I can go through an exercise routine and do the other things I do, but changing the bed destroys my saturation. That triggers an emotional response in many of us. "Life is over. I cannot even make the bed." My solution was to surrender. I keep the bed made and sleep on top of it with a couple of fluffy throws. They go in the wash every couple of days, the top blanket goes in the wash once a week. (Remember – fine particulate matter is your enemy.)*

51)   *Predators. There are people out there looking to prey on desperate people. Before setting up a payment plan for several thousand dollars, talk to your doctor. Read Yelp reviews. Look at the fine print. They usually promise a miracle cure, and in the fine print say:*

These statements have not been evaluated by the Food and Drug Administration. This information is not intended to suggest diagnosis, treatment, cure or prevention of any disease.

Ask them to show their randomized controlled trials in patients with COPD. (You do not need to know what that means.) They will not be able to. If they show you a study done by one person who was not vetted for conflict of interest, it is not a legitimate study.

52)   *This pillow is a straight-up miracle. They are losing a wide market by calling it a pregnancy pillow. It supports every part of your body and keeps you in the position that is optimal for you.*

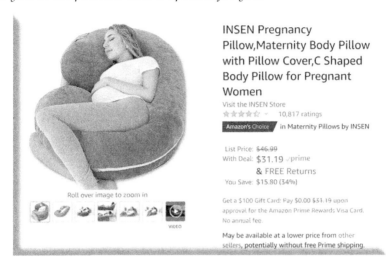

53)   *Lastly – COMPUTER SAFETY. We are telling you to Google things and giving you links. If the words "Privacy Policy" appear on a site that you are on, that means they are gathering and selling data they find in your computer or phone.*

It is a good idea to purchase Malwarebytes, or get the free version and run it periodically, or purchase Norton 360. This will confuse the data-gathering programs trying to find their way into your device. If you are computer savvy, browsers usually have add-ons which will protect your privacy.

NEVER click on an unknown link. Law enforcement has not caught up to technology. People can download malware into your computer that will record keystrokes and gather passwords and banking information.

***

COPD Hacks and Tricks will be updated periodically. When one of us learns something, we all learn something. For the latest version please visit our website.

If you are reading an electronic version of this book you can click on https://thesecrettothrivingwithcopd.com.

If you are reading a paper copy, enter thesercrettothrivingwithcopd.com in the browser of your computer.

PLEASE FEEL FREE TO PASS THIS ON.

.

***

REHAB

Moving around, safely, is the single most important thing you can do to stay healthy.

Ask your doctor if pulmonary rehabilitation is available. If you can find a respiratory therapist or a physiotherapist, you have struck gold. To our great fortune, we have a few of them hanging out on our site.

Following will be links to Rachel Garrod's page and exercise videos. I asked Rachel, a physiotherapist, the exercises she considered the most important. Chair stands, because they enable you to move around. If the chair stands are too difficult, you can stack books on the chair to raise it. Simply sit on the chair, cross your arms, and stand up. Shoulder sweeps (slowly pull your arms and shoulders back, like rowing a boat), because they allow your lungs to expand. Put a balance exercise in there.

All these exercises are in the videos at the bottom of the page.

There is also a free Pulmonary Rehab bootcamp on Facebook:

https://www.facebook.com/groups/UltimatePulmonaryWellness/

You can incorporate rehab into your life just by doing things, pushing yourself a little. I do not do things that I know are going to tank my saturation, but I walk the track at the dog park, get out there and work in the garden, and wrestle around with my dogs. The more you move, the more you will want to move. When I am exhausted, I exercise. Five minutes into stretching and toning, the exhaustion lifts.

Rachel has a plethora of free stuff on her page, as well as an option to pay 45 American dollars or 300 euros for a one-on-one Messenger or Skype session.

Remember: you do not have superpowers on Prednisone. Jumping off the roof, thinking you can fly, is not recommended.

Rachel Garrod's page (make sure and scroll through – there is a LOT of stuff in there)

https://www.facebook.com/rachelgarrodphysio/

Always *have a chair with you. If you need to exercise sitting down, sit down. If it hurts**, stop**. Do not do that exercise or do a modified version.*

What you feed grows. Or the wolf you feed is the wolf who wins. You can say it a million different ways – the theory is the same. If you start moving around, just a little, it will snowball.

Do not overdo it, especially if you are on Prednisone.

*Start slow. Try a chair stand. Pull your shoulders back with your elbows and hold for a moment. It opens your airways, and it **feels** good.*

You can find exercise videos and a guided meditation Rachel does on https://thesecrettothrivingwithcopd.com.

EXERCISE

O *ur bodies crave movement. From the time we develop limbs in the womb we are thrashing around. We emerge into the world, take that first magic breathe, and go into motion.*

Kids are unstoppable.

When we age some of us become sedentary. The less one moves, the less one wants to move.

Energy begets energy.

My dad exercised every morning. I thought it was weird. Okay, but weird.

The man had energy. He was as active at eighty as he was at fifty. Retirement was not a thing for Dad. He was also unstoppable.

My mom tried to take his ladders away when he broke six ribs and his clavicle falling off a ladder. He kept a sneaky folding ladder in the trunk of his car. He was still whipping that ladder out at eighty years old.

A blood thinner took him down at eighty-four. It was an exceptionally vigorous eighty-four. When my mom died, he moved in with me. At one point he was dating three women, one a stripper named Candi.

My brother said he felt like he was raising a teenager.

Sel says that if he dies at eighty-four, he hopes someone must get rid of his condoms before the relatives show up.

During the pandemic I had new a lot of healthy people who felt awful. They had quit moving around. As the months wore on, they became used to being sedentary.

Again, the less one moves, the less one wants to move.

I was working on this book with Rachel. As she explained why exercise worked, I took more of an interest in exercise. The more I exercised the better I felt.

I remember Bethany, from rehab, telling me that when she missed a day, she felt it.

Strong muscles ask for less oxygen.

The dog park was my salvation during the pandemic. The dogs and I got cardio walking the track. With Camden, our two-year-old tripod, I get a lot of cardio. Camden thinks that dogs with four legs are weird.

People who did not walk the track I watched struggle.

Pre-rehab, I was one of those people who wondered why on earth people wanted to lift weights. They are heavy.

Not that our rehab weights are that heavy. I use four-pound weights I got from Amazon. Unless you already have arm strength, I would recommend starting out with one or two-pound weights.

You do not even have to use weights. They give the exercise added impact, but you can just clench your fists. Or, use a couple of cans of soup.

***

THREE IMPORTANT THINGS

1) **Check with your doctor before undertaking anything strenuous.**

2) **If it hurts, STOP. Do not do that exercise or do a modified version. You can do most of these exercises sitting in a chair.**

3) *ALWAYS have a chair with you. If you want to sit down, sit down.*

Until you know how balanced you are, keep one hand on the back of the chair. During balance exercises, keep your hand over the back of the chair so you can grab it.

***

Rachel and I both have exercises on YouTube. You can get to them on our website, https://thesecrettothrivingwithcopd.com.

There are a lot of COPD exercises on YouTube. There is also a free online pulmonary rehab boot camp link in the Tricks and Hacks chapter.

Find the ones you like.

In addition to giving me a life, exercise has reduced my pain level.

I qualified for a knew replacement a long time ago, but I am leery of the downtime. I cannot be put out because my lung function is too low, but I have had surgery with local anesthetic.

(I crushed my wrist when I tripped getting out of a rental SUV that should have had an extension ladder to climb down. I spent a couple of hours listening to the surgeons say things like "Maybe if we put this one here, that can go there."

The anesthesiologist was the only one who knew I was awake. My head was tented. One surgeon said, "How does someone not know the depth of their own step?"

I said, "When they are in a freaking rental."

*It was quiet for quite a while. Finally, in a small voice, "Well they usually do not talk back **during** surgery.")*

I also have a herniated disc in my neck that makes itself known.

I have learned stretches that keep the pain quiet enough that I rarely think of it. Unless I go a couple of days without exercising.

Our exercise physiologist says, "Motion is lotion." It truly is. When I do not exercise, I creak and groan like the Tin Man in the Wizard of Oz.

Start slow.

Pace yourself.

Do a couple of simple exercises. Take a break. Do one more.

Go at your pace. You can go through a routine every day, or you can take a few moments and do the exercises that make you feel better.

Fatigue is a huge component of this disease. We have gone through the "The less you move, the less you want to move" thing.

The opposite holds true. Energy begets energy. The more you move, the more you want to move.

I go through a routine three times a week and do the important ones every day.

Chair stands and shoulder rolls.

I get cardio at the dog park and now on the Nu-Step at rehab.

There are not many of us that have ongoing pulmonary rehabilitation available. For those of us lucky enough to have a group, we lost that group during the pandemic.

I had Rachel Garrod, explaining how exercise battles back weakness, breathlessness, and fatigue.

So, I exercised. For the most part. I got lazy once, and I got depressed and lazy once more. I got weak in a hurry. Weak enough to get scared, and to grab my weights.

I have friends who lost rehab during the pandemic that got so weak they ended up in the hospital.

They are still trying to come back from it. I remember Bethany telling me years ago that when she missed a day at rehab, she felt it.

It would be great if we all had a group. Hopefully, the decision makers will someday realize that pulmonary rehabilitation keeps us out of the hospital and offer it to everyone who is willing to put the effort into themselves.

Again, pulmonary rehabilitation is cheap, effective medicine.

You will not turn into the Energizer Bunny the first time you exercise.

You will slowly but surely strengthen your muscles. Talk to your doctor and make sure your heart is okay and do something for cardio. Walking. Dancing. Swimming.

Gradually you will find yourself less breathless and have more energy.

Rachel told me that she considered shoulder rolls and chair stands to be two crucial exercises, so I will start with those.

As I said before, you can use weights, cans of soup, or just keep your hands fisted. I use four-pound (1.8 KG) weights that I got from Amazon, but I worked up to four pounds. Unless you already have arm strength, start with something smaller.

(Elizabeth works with twelve-pound weights (5.4 KG). I think she is one of those people that can lift cars off children.)

I must offer a disclaimer on the exercise drawings. They are not drawn to scale and your limbs will not bend in the manner of the limbs of the little exercise people. These drawings are to give you an understanding of the movement. They are not portraits.

Portraits would have taken an extraordinary amount of time.

Shoulder rolls are important for three reasons. They open your airways, making it easier to breathe. They improve your posture. When you are slumped over, it is difficult to breathe. And, they just plain feel good.

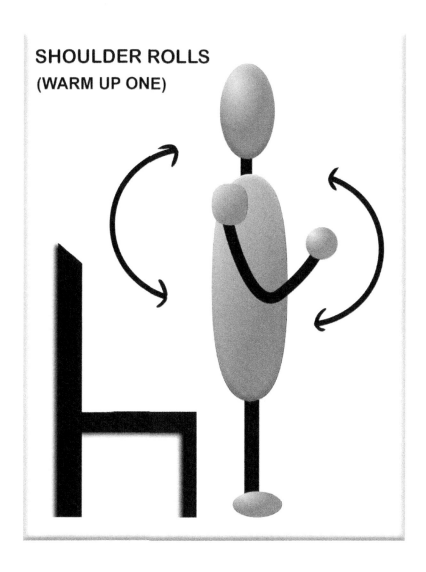

SHOULDER ROLLS
(WARM UP ONE)

Bring your hands up and roll your shoulders backwards. Gently squeeze your shoulder blades together. Move in large, slow circles.

Ten repetitions. Eventually.

This is a warm-up exercise. I am going out of order with the chair stands because if you can only manage to do two exercises a day some days, these are the ones you want to do.

If you like, you can hold on to weights for added impact to the shoulder rolls. Do a few without weights to warm up, then add the weights.

Chair stands are the other exercise I do every day.

When I came to rehab, I never knew if I would be able to make it across the room or not. A common complaint from those of us in the lower stages is "I cannot even make it to the mailbox any longer!"

Chair stands will strengthen your legs and enable you to move about the world again.

Simply sit in a chair. Cross your arms or grasp your elbows. Stand up.

If standing from a seated position is too difficult at first, you can stack books on the chair to make it easier. As it gets easier, remove one book at a time.

Chair Stand Begin

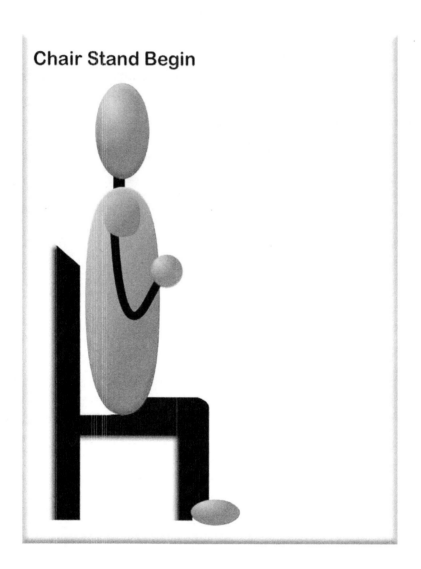

Chair Stand Movement

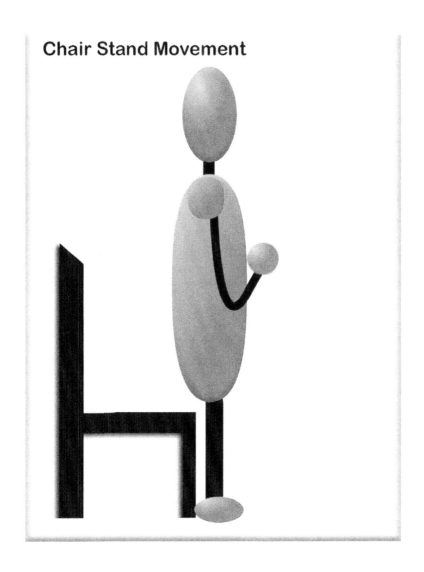

You have taken a step towards improving your health.

That is powerful.

Ten repetitions a day. Eventually.

You know your body. We will give you a few exercises. Search on YouTube for COPD exercises to find out if there are exercises more suited to you.

Again, check with your doctor before undertaking anything strenuous. Make sure that your heat is okay. If you have cardiac issues, find out if cardiac rehabilitation is available.

You can build your own routine or follow along with Rachel or me on YouTube.

Or – simply move around. As Rachel says, do what you love, but move.

Ask your doctor if pulmonary rehabilitation is available to you. If you can find a rehab specialist, you have struck gold.

Groups are great. Many people found it tough to keep going without a group during the pandemic. Thank the fates, I had a Rachel Garrod.

As things stand now in the U.S., Medicare will only pay for seventy-two visits.

We are hoping that changes.

Add your voice. Make it clear to your doctor that you want rehab, that you want to thrive, that expensive inhalers and blowing in a tube once a year are not cutting it.

Tell your doctor that exhaustive research has proven pulmonary rehabilitation to be cheap medicine that works.

If we all had pulmonary rehab maintenance available, if we all had a group run by rehab professionals to go to, pulmonary medicine would change.

Far less time would be spent in the hospital. Again, because I have a group, I have never been hospitalized.

Those of us in the lower stages would be able to make it across the room, then to the mailbox, then to the dog park or the mall.

Those of us in the upper stages would not live in fear of slipping into the lower stages.

Build your routine, whatever it is. Do it two or three times a week. Add something for cardio, after you have talked to your doctor. If you like to dance, turn up the music and move.

Warm up – if you are beginning a routine, do the shoulder rolls without weights as Warm Up One.

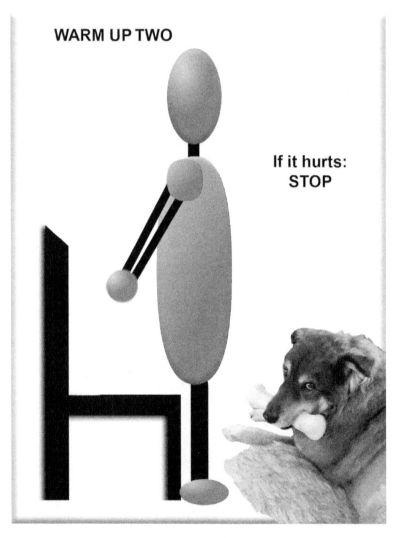

Clasp your hands behind you and **gently** raise your arms until you feel a stretch. Hold for ten seconds.

I do this every morning. It is a great stretch.

WARM UP THREE

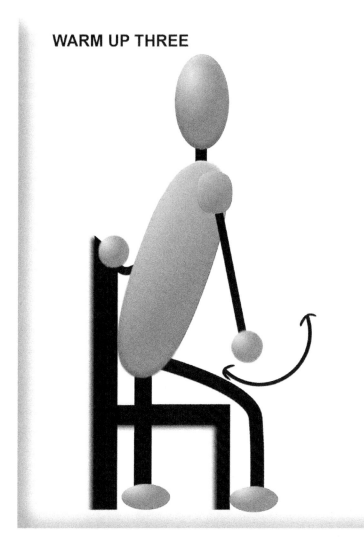

Lean forward, resting one arm on the back of your chair or your knee.

Let your other arm hang loose. Swing it in large, slow circles. Five repetitions one way, then change direction, five more repetitions.

Repeat with your other arm.

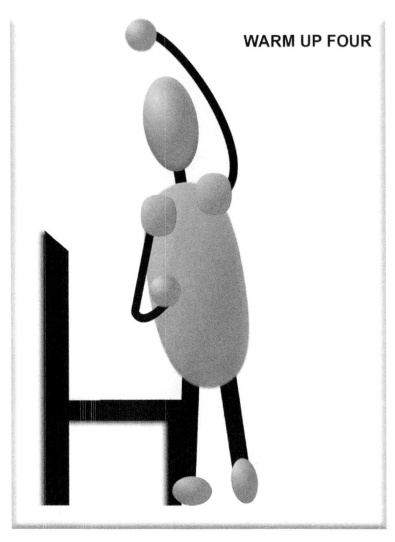

Lean to one side and stretch one arm over your head, towards the side in which you are leaning, until you feel a stretch. Lean to the other side and stretch in the opposite direction with your other arm. Ten repetitions.

WARM UP FIVE

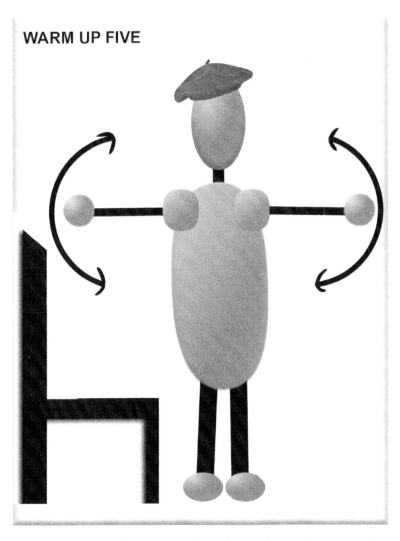

Hold your arms straight out to the sides and gently move them in a windmill motion. Large, loose circles. Five forward, five backwards.

This one took me off the knee replacement list. Motion is lotion, indeed.

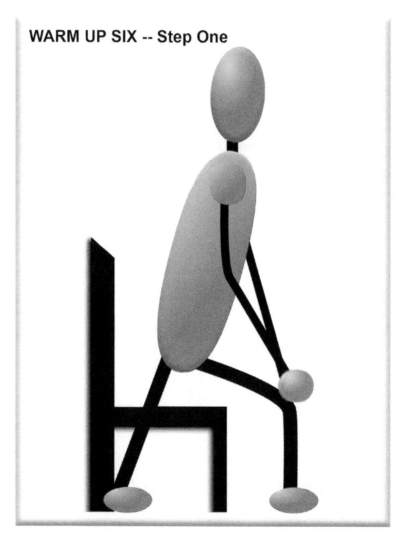

WARM UP SIX -- Step One

Lean forward until you feel a stretch in your back leg. You can keep one hand on the back of your chair, or if you are comfortable with your balance, place both hands on your front knee. Hold for a count of five.

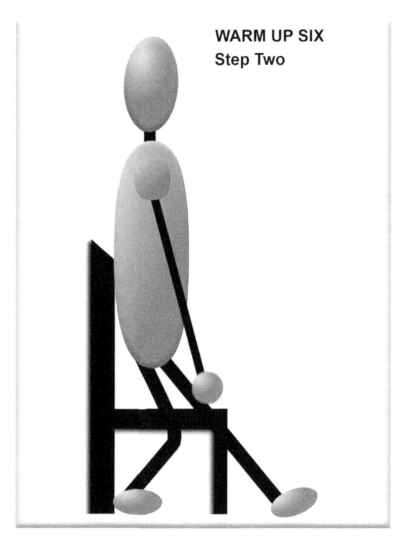

WARM UP SIX
Step Two

Shift your weight to your back leg, bending your back knee, until you feel a stretch in your front leg. Tilt your front foot up. You can hold onto your chair, or place both hands on your front knee if you are comfortable with your balance. Hold for a count of five.

Repeat the whole thing using your other leg.

This is the point at which you will do your chair stands. Sit in a chair. Cross your arms in front of you or grasp your elbows. Stand.

If it is too difficult, stack books in the chair to make it easier. Start with two or three chair stands. Gradually remove one book at a time and add another chair stand until you can do ten.

Exhausting yourself the first time you exercise is **not** the goal here.

The goal is to **gradually** strengthen your muscles.

As I said before, one measure they use to define how damaged you are is "tolerance to exercise".

As you increase your exercise tolerance you become less damaged.

Movement is magic.

While you are sitting in the chair, you might as well do a great core exercise. Core exercises strengthen muscles that aid your lungs and help gain control of a large belly. If you are overweight, it will be harder to breathe. Your belly is pressuring your diaphragm, the bellows system that draws in breath.

Being underweight can also be a problem. Core exercises will not keep you from gaining weight if you are trying to gain weight. They will simply strengthen muscles that aid in breathing.

Strengthening your core muscles leads to better balance and stability. Weak core muscles can lead to fatigue and loss of endurance.

EXERCISE TWO

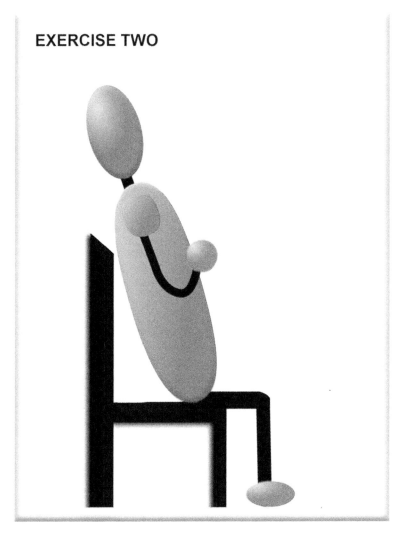

Sit on the edge of your chair with your arms crossed in front of you. Lean back, stop just before your back touches the chair. Hold for a count of five.

10 repetitions. Eventually.

If there is no pain, *you can add a twist to the left, then to the right.*

EXERCISE THREE

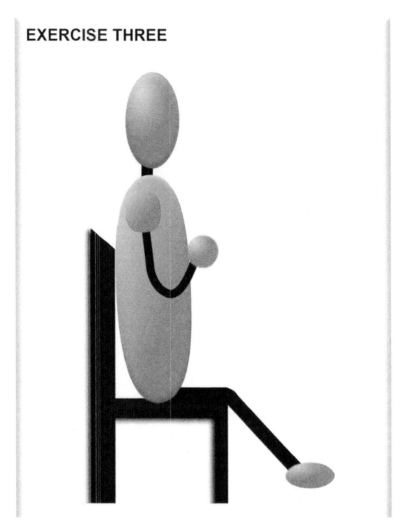

This is another core exercise, strengthening your abdominal muscles and building endurance.

Sit in your chair and lift your legs. The level of difficulty is up to you. You can lift them just a bit, or you can stretch them strait out in front of you. Start with just a bit. Hold for a count of three to five.

EXERCISE FOUR

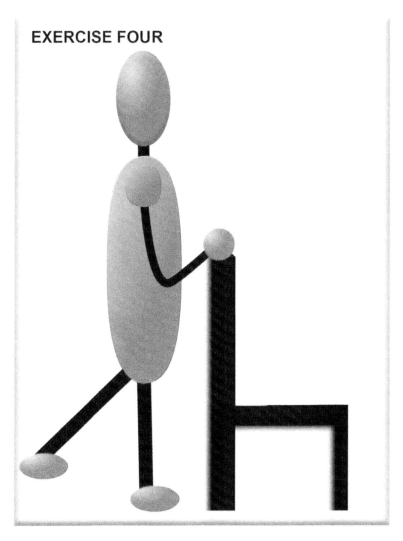

This one performs double duty as a core exercise and an upper leg stretch. Stand behind your chair with your hands on back of the chair. Lift one leg up. Hold for a count of three to five.

Repeat with other leg.

EXERCISE FIVE
Knee Raises

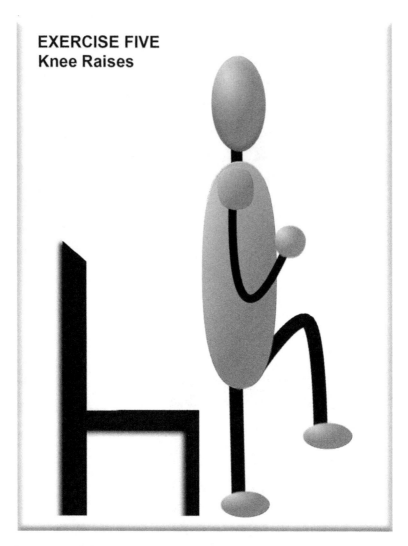

March in place, lifting your knee up high.

Twelve repetitions.

OR

If you wish to add difficulty you can work your arms and legs at the same time.

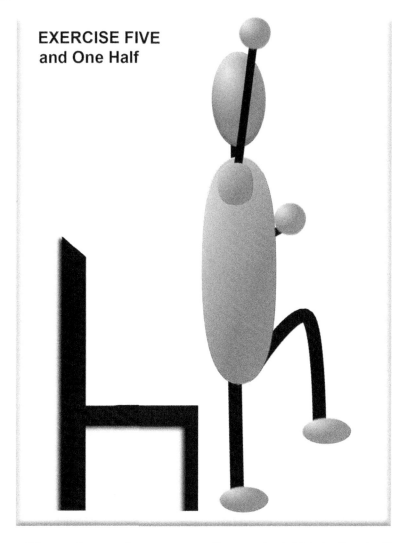

EXERCISE FIVE and One Half

As you lift your knee, raise your opposite arm straight into the air. Repeat with your other leg and your other arm. (It will take a minute for your body to figure this one out.)

Ten repetitions.

EXERCISE SIX
Side Leg Raises

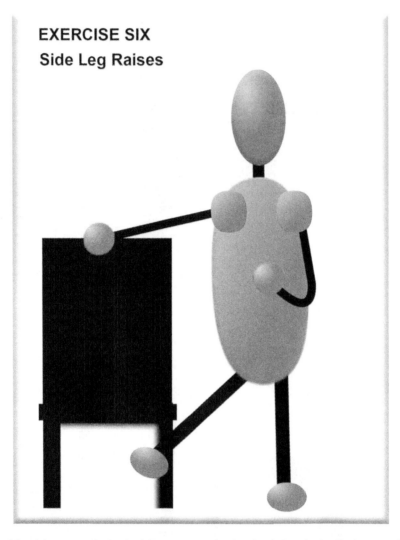

Stand beside your chair, holding on to the back of the chair. Raise one leg to the side, bring it back down and lift the other.

Ten repetitions.

Balance is huge. Any good doctor will tell you the secret to a long life and good health is "Don't fall."

Healthy people break things and end up with pneumonia from being bedridden. We cannot afford to break things.

I had no idea how unbalanced I was until I tried to do a balance exercise. "Try" is the operative word here. It took a while before I could stay balanced for a count of one.

Always *keep your hand just above the top of your chair. You will be grabbing it a lot at first.*

EXERCISE SEVEN
Balance

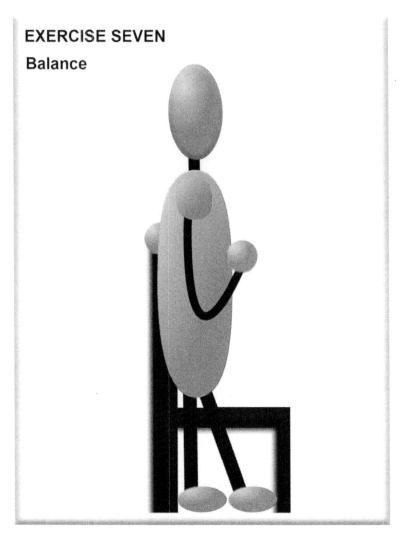

Holding onto the back of your chair, place one foot directly in front of the other. Lift your hand above the chair. Eventually you will be able to hold for a count of ten without grabbing the chair.

Repeat with other foot.

EXERCISE EIGHT
Balance

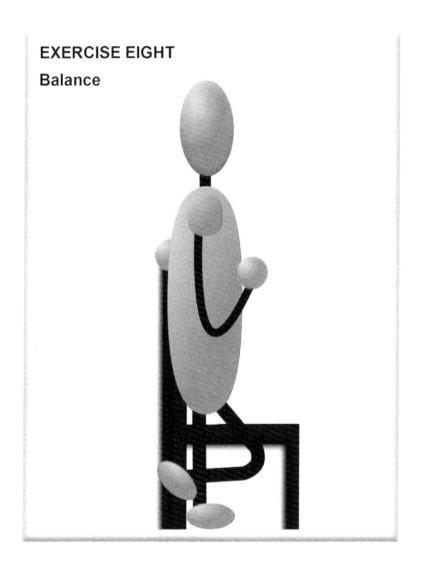

Holding onto the back of your chair, lift one foot. You can hold it any way you like – I tuck mine behind my other leg.

Lift your hand from the chair, keeping it just above the back of the chair.

Eventually you will be able to hold for a count of ten.

Repeat with other foot.

Arm strength and Posture.

Your posture is huge when it comes to breathing. When our shoulders are slumped, we are compromising our ability to fill our lungs. The better your posture the easier it is to breathe.

Arm strength may not seem like a big deal, but we use our arms for just about everything. If the muscles in our arms are weak, we tire quickly. We then fall into the cycle of "the less you move, the less you want to move". If we quit moving it does not take long to become weak.

We are a bit like sharks. They must be in motion.

Two weeks *of not exercising had me convinced I was dying. I felt damaged, as though I was slipping into a deeper stage of this disease.*

It took a month of exercise to start feeling strong again.

Most people with my lung function are in wheelchairs. I would be if Patrick Moan had not talked me into fighting for pulmonary rehabilitation. If I was still alive.

I just went up to five-pound weights. Sel called and told me here were weights on sale at a store he was at.

I said, "I think I am good with the four-pounds."

Silence. More silence.

I went up to five pounds. Stronger is better. Elizabeth told me to decrease the repetitions for a bit.

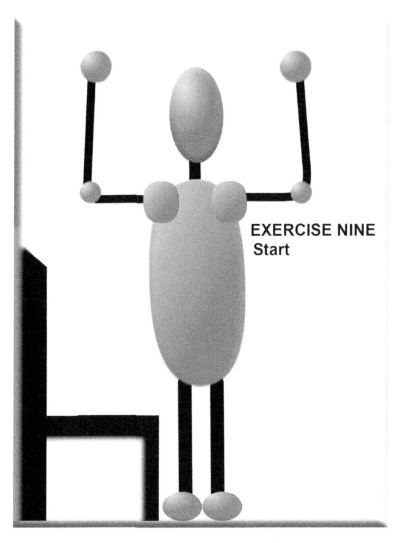

EXERCISE NINE
Start

Start with your arms out to the side, bent at the elbow, your hands straight up. With or without weights.

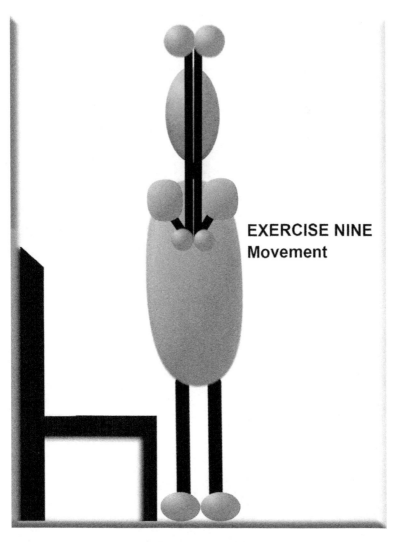

EXERCISE NINE
Movement

Keeping your upper and lower arms at a right angle, bring your elbows and hands together.

Nine Repetitions.

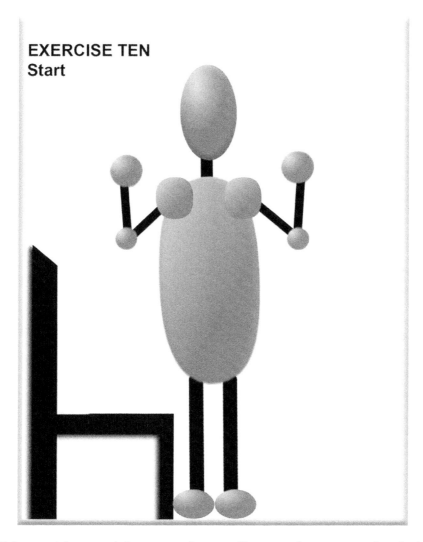

EXERCISE TEN
Start

With or without weights, extend your elbows and arms out, hands just above shoulder height.

Remember to keep your back straight.

Push your hands up in the air.

173

EXERCISE TEN Movement

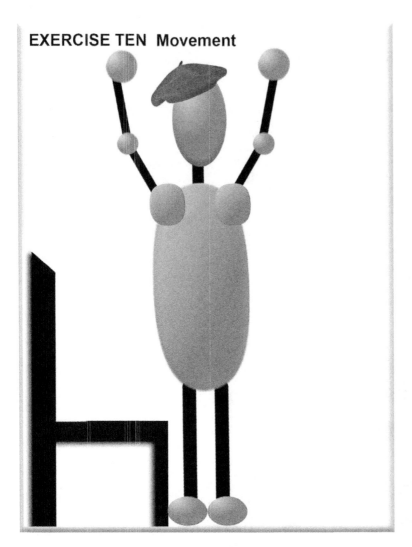

Ten repetitions.

Start with your arms hanging straight down, with or without weights.

(Are you keeping your back straight?)

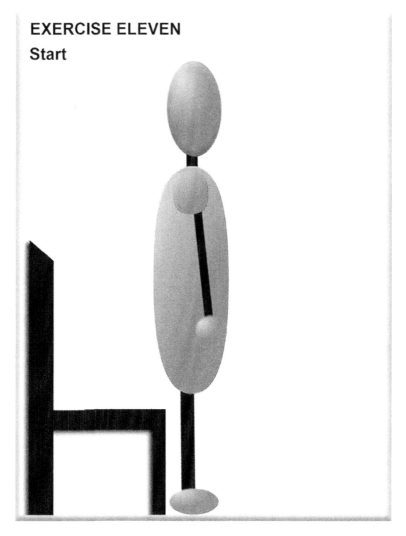

EXERCISE ELEVEN
Start

Keeping your upper arm straight, curl your lower arm and your hand to your chest, with or without weights.

EXERCISE ELEVEN
Movement

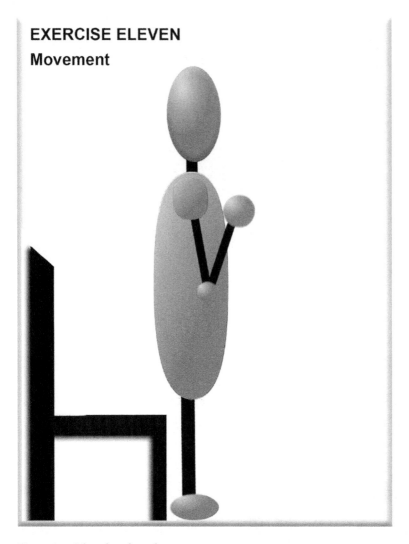

Repeat with other hand.

Ten repetitions.

*This is a **great** exercise. It has the benefit of being easy and low impact while strengthening several parts of your body and improving your posture.*

It strengthens your back, your abdominal muscles, your upper arms, and your upper legs.

EXERCISE TWELVE
Start

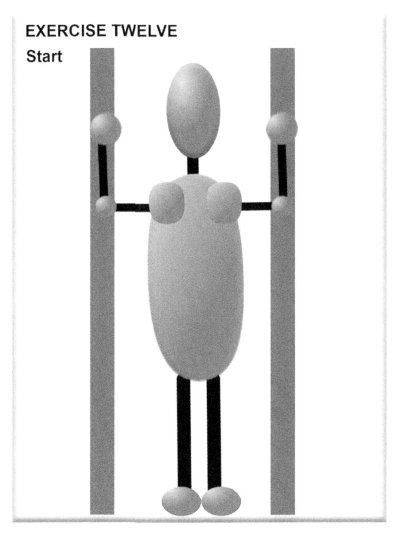

Stand facing a doorway, your upper arms placed on either side of the door jam.

EXERCISE TWELVE Movement

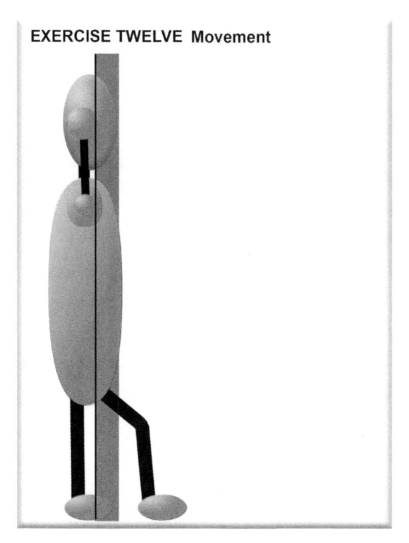

Place one foot through the doorway.

Hold for a count of five.

Ten repetitions.

Cool down. (I know, right? More exercises.)

COOL DOWN ONE

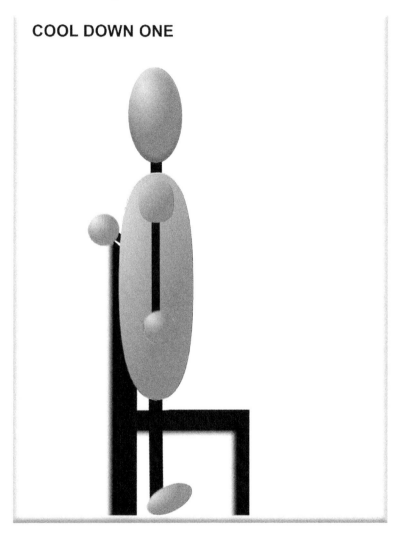

Hold on to the back of your chair – this is also a balance exercise.

Rock back and forth from your heels to your toes.

COOL DOWN ONE Step Two

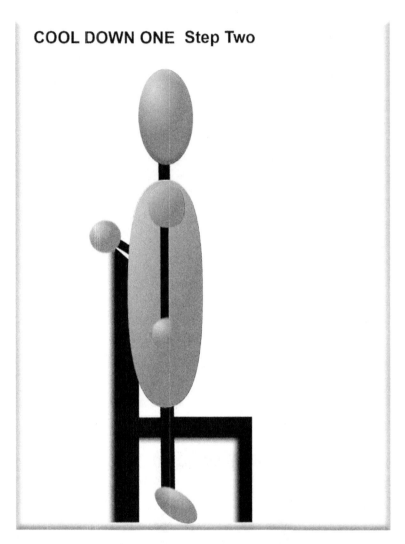

Ten repetitions.

COOL DOWN TWO

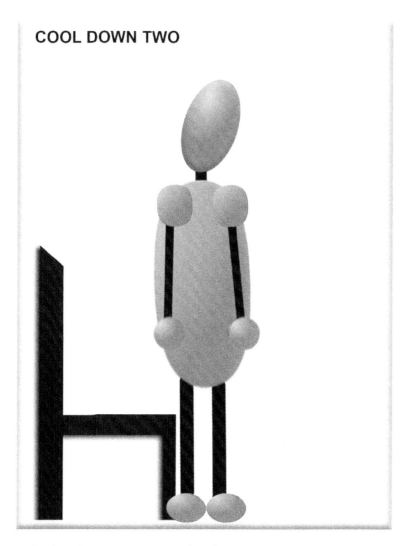

IF IT DOES NOT HURT – *Gently tilt your head to one side until you feel a stretch. Hold for a count of ten.*

Repeat, holding your head to the other side.

COOL DOWN THREE

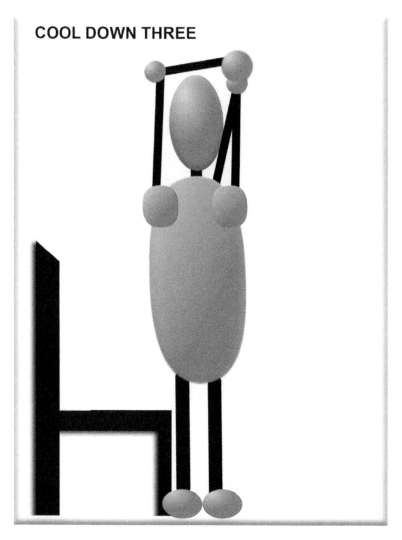

Lift your left arm up and place your left hand behind you, between your shoulder blades. Grasp your left elbow with your right hand and gently pull your left arm back until you feel a stretch.

Hold for ten seconds.

Repeat with other arm.

Hold onto the back of your chair. Left your right foot up behind you with your right hand, gently, until you feel a stretch.

Do not let yourself become frustrated if you cannot lift your leg remarkably high. Flexibility comes with time. I can pull my foot up to my back – now. It took time to get there.

Hold for a count of ten. Eventually. Repeat with other leg.

My body is flexible because I exercise at least three times a week. I shoot for
a   few   exercises   eve

COOL DOWN FOUR

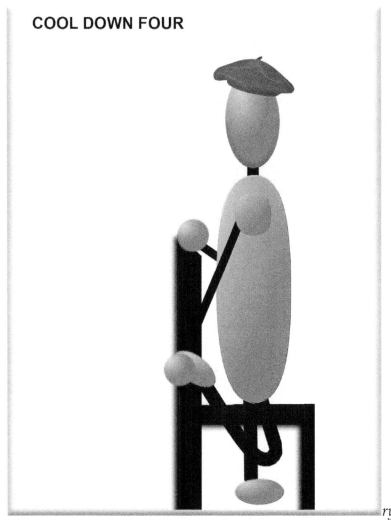

ry day, and I go through my routine three times a week.

I get cardio at the dog park.

When you gain flexibility, you lose pain. I have found a stretch to conquer everything that causes me pain.

I have several serious issues and I have not taken so much as a Tylenol in months.

184

If you have done these exercises, or your version of these exercises, you have improved your health.

Every single time you exercise you improve your health.

You probably do not feel like exercising. Like me, six years ago, you may not be able to successfully walk across the room.

The human body craves movement. When you give it a little movement, your body gives you energy for more movement.

Rachel helps people with COPD learn to thrive for a living. I am a living testament to the power of Pulmonary Rehabilitation.

You do not have to believe rehab works because we are saying it works. International Task Forces and several hundred studies have proved that pulmonary rehabilitation works, no matter what stage you are at.

You have exercised! You have reason to be proud of yourself. Keep it up. Six weeks from now, stop and think about how you felt six weeks ago.

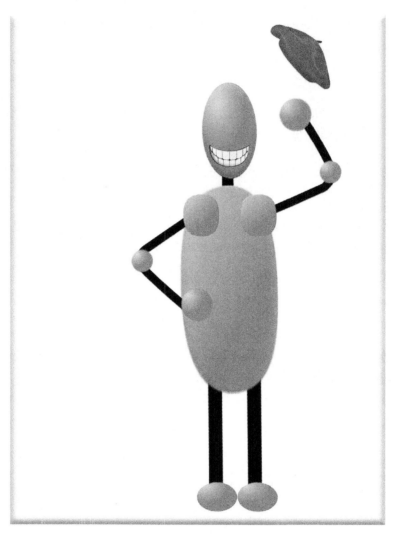

You will be amazed. That is a promise.

WHY IS PULMONARY REHABILITATION BEING WITHHELD?

*P*ulmonary rehabilitation has proven to be cheap medicine that works. Period.

*The shame of this whole thing is that it **is** a secret, withheld from so many people.*

This should be shouted from rooftops.

Why is this life changing treatment not available to everyone who wants it?

Currently the U.S. spends almost fifty billion dollars a year on COPD, mostly on hospital stays.

Due to rehab, I have not once been hospitalized.

Studies prove that pulmonary rehabilitation reduces hospital readmissions. Despite this, ongoing rehab is available to virtually no one, and when it is available, it is often denied to fourth stage patients.

I tell people in the upper three stages "If they could bring me back from the dead, they can turn you into Spider Man." (Gender politics aside.)

When I found out that rehab worked even in patients as "far gone" as I, I thought the PMA would surely want to know.

The PMA did not want to know.

I wrote a lengthy letter. No response. I called and asked to speak to the manager. She said she had received the letter and given it "to someone".

That was it.

I wrote them another lengthy letter.

No response.

I started writing lengthy letters to **everyone**. *Anyone who had something to do with pulmonary medicine and had an email or a mailing address got a letter.*

I heard from several people who said that rehab had been keeping them alive decades past their "die by" date, but only because they had good insurance. One by one, they told me they did not know why pulmonary medicine in this country did not pay attention to studies and told me to try the next organization on my list.

The last letter I wrote was to Medicare. I thought surely, they would want to do the math.

Medicare did not want to do the math. I got a curt response telling me "There is protocol for pulmonary rehabilitation, and you are the exception to the rule."

I know a great many "exceptions to the rule" who would disagree with them.

I drew the line at writing to AARP. I got as far as getting a membership.

I met with a book club that was discussing the autobiography I wrote. We mostly talked about dogs. There is indeed bank robbery and many spectacularly bad life choices, but the book turned into a love story about dogs.

Rick had gone with me. He told me, "You should write a book about COPD."

Rick had been there when I got the death sentence. Rick had watched me come back from the dead, cheering me on. He lives in a houseboat he built himself, on the river – he drives all the way across town to hang out at the dog park with me and my pack.

I automatically said, "I am working on something else."

Speculative fiction is my first love. I officially have a junior high school education, having left home so young. I am a reader, though. Through reading, I continue to give myself a world-class education.

The lessons that stick with me are slipped through the back door of my mind while I am reading for entertainment. I had no idea that I had internalized Plato at nine-years-old, reading the Chronicles of Narnia, until I took a community college philosophy course.

(I did take the fun stuff in college.)

My epic philosophy teacher was talking about Plato's "Allegory of the Cave". I raised my hand and recited a Narnia line:

"Their prison is only in their minds, yet they are in that prison, and so afraid of being taken in that they cannot be taken out."

My professor's eyes flashed, he pointed at me, and thundered "EXACTLY!"

I have learned things of great import reading speculative fiction, and I have had a book writing itself in my head for a long time.

I thought about it when I got home.

I had been writing letters for three years. With letters to Medicare and pulmonary medicine, I was shouting in the wind.

With letters to people who deal with real life COPD, I was preaching to the choir.

None of it was effective.

I deleted to beginnings of the AARP letter and started to write a book.

To my great joy, a physiotherapist who hangs out on the COPD site just for the sake of helping people agreed to collaborate with me.

Rachel is wicked smart. When I started hunting for studies on pulmonary rehabilitation, she sent me dozens of them. She had taken part in most of them.

Rachel also has a gorgeous voice with a British accent – listen to her guided meditation.

*The COPD related healthcare costs for 2020 in the United States has not been calculated yet, but it was projected to hit forty-nine **billion** dollars. Most of that is hospital costs. Medicare and Medicaid bear the brunt of the cost – private insurance pays for around eighteen percent.*

In Northern California, the average COPD related hospital stay costs $80,818. If the ICU is involved, which it often is, that number jumps to $144,318. *UC Davis Transparency Master

Again, I have never been hospitalized. This is a direct result of pulmonary rehabilitation. I exercise and stay strong enough to stay out of the hospital. The women at rehab have taught me how to monitor my health so I can catch something early that might turn out to be hospital-worthy for people who do not take their measurements.

I have no idea how much a pulmonary rehabilitation program cost. I suspect it is a small fraction of what is spent on hospitalizations.

I read through studies until my eyes glazed. There have been countless studies on pulmonary rehabilitation. There are three findings that run through all of them.

1) *Reduced dypsnea. (Shortness of breath.)*
2) *Reduced mortality rates.*
3) *Reduced healthcare costs. Reduced hospital admissions/readmissions.*

*Those three alone are huge. That is what COPD **is**. Breathlessness, hospitalization, death.*

*A program of targeted exercise is **the** answer.*

Besides the whole keeping-people-alive thing, ongoing pulmonary rehabilitation slashes healthcare costs.

These are not a few small, random studies.

In 2013 there was a joint Task Force, the British Lung Foundation, and the American Thoracic Society, which cited over three hundred studies and involved forty-nine vetted medical professionals.

These people went over every piece of data they could find on pulmonary rehabilitation and its' effect on the patient and healthcare.

This was their major finding and recommendation:

Embedding pulmonary rehabilitation concepts into the evidence-based management of respiratory disease

Given the overwhelming effect of pulmonary rehabilitation, it is important that the service can be made available to as many patients in need of it as possible. This requires the need for programmes that are within the reach for patients and referring physicians that are adequately referring to these programmes. Legislators should consider making pulmonary rehabilitation mandatory prior to or in the context of other expensive healthcare interventions are considered for patients (e.g. expensive pharmacotherapy for dedicated respiratory diseases and surgical procedures) or when patients were hospitalized for their respiratory disease.

In summary, the future of pulmonary rehabilitation is bright. The future of rehabilitation is geared towards engaging more patients in better tailored programmes. To that end, programmes need to

be widely advertised, and healthcare professionals need to be well trained to deal with the individual needs and preferences of patients. Exercise therapy should be seen as an individualized programme on the edge of patient's capacities in order to provide an as potent as possible training stimulus. Towards the end of the programme, patients need to develop self-management skills that allow them to deal with their disease, maintain the benefits of the programme and translate them into enhanced quality and quantity of physical activity.

It does not get much clearer than that. Pulmonary rehabilitation should be integrated into pulmonary medicine and offered to as many people as possible.

That has not happened. Rehab is largely not available, and when it is it is often denied to those in the lower stages, the people who have the most to gain from rehab.

Just recently I realized that I had never seen a Medicare bill from rehab. I asked about it. I was stunned when the rehab director told me that Medicare does not pay for ongoing rehab.

The healthcare system I am in pays for ongoing pulmonary rehabilitation themselves, with a small copay.

I did not realize how fortunate I was.

Medicare gets it right with the machines. The woman from Medicare who helped me get the Life2000 could not have been more helpful.

Whoever oversees pulmonary rehabilitation has not taken a close look at research for an exceptionally long time, though.

Kind of like veterinarians who still think that hormones are good for dogs.

Medicare sets the stage in the U.S. for medical treatment. Many doctors just follow along.

*Thank the fates for my healthcare system, who realized that rehab keeps COPD patients out of the hospital, and cares enough to **want** to keep us out of the hospital.*

People want rehab. If ongoing pulmonary rehabilitation were available to everyone who wanted it, pulmonary medicine would look much, much different.

Not everyone has the discipline to exercise at home. Sometimes I do not have the discipline to exercise at home. Being able to go in once a week has been my lifeline.

Some people need to exercise in a safe setting. We have people in our group who want to go to the gym, and whose doctors are telling them that they should not exercise alone. They have already used up all the rehab that Medicare will pay for, though, so…….

So….what? Do not exercise, become weak, slip into the lower stages of this disease.

That is not necessary.

Ongoing pulmonary rehabilitation. Reduced breathlessness. Quality of life. Not visiting home briefly between hospital stays – staying home.

Outliving your dogs.

I am not the exception to the rule. I was willing to do the work, and my healthcare system gave me people who showed me what the work is. Even though I "did not meet protocol."

This is a win/win. Some people do not want to put in the work. Okay.

For those that do, ongoing pulmonary rehabilitation should be an absolute right.

What is the problem here?

Denying ongoing pulmonary rehabilitation to pulmonary patients is akin to denying antibiotics to patients with a mild systemic infection.

"Come back when you are septic and need to be hospitalized."

I am not so naive that I do not know there are people on the other end of that cash flow who are satisfied with the status quo, the $485 inhalers, the $80,000 to $144,000 hospital stays.

That cannot be the entirety of pulmonary medicine, though.

The healthcare system I am in has treated me exceptionally well, apart from that first diagnosing doctor and the nurse practitioners who worked under him.

"No. You are too sick to exercise. Just turn your oxygen all the way up — so you are comfortable."

Once I got past that hurdle, I found a system that takes care of its' people.

I joined the ZDoggMD Supporter Tribe to try and figure out how healthcare works. I am no closer to figuring out how healthcare works, but I found an entire tribe of medical professionals who are passionate about healthcare. Dr. Z and his Tribe have the triple trifecta going on: smart, funny, and conscious. They are among the best of medicine.

*Dr. Z himself is like a new superhero. Instead of leaping tall buildings in a single bound, he lasers through medical chaos and red tape and relentlessly **makes sense**.*

I have heard stories about for-profit hospitals that would earn the praise of any evil James Bond villain. The lengths they will go to for money are hard to credit, until you see the paperwork.

We still have the old guard pulmonologists, who quit looking at studies sometime around the turn of the century and believe that sick people should not exercise.

I keep thinking of Rachel, all those years ago, sneaking pulmonary patients out for exercise, only to get busted by panicked nurses.

"Stop that this instant! That patient needs to be in bed!"

Some people, as I said, do not want to do the work. I joined a fourth stage group to see what they were up to.

Nothing. They were up to nothing. They welcomed each other home from the hospital. I started talking about rehab and they threw me out.

"Leave us alone! We are dying!"

If not for the dogs, I probably would have been one of those people. I cannot die on my dogs.

Ongoing pulmonary rehabilitation also must have minimum standards. We have members who have heard all this great stuff about rehab. They find out it is available to them and get a referral. When they show up, someone points at the machines and tells them to have fun.

I do not know what to call that. You cannot call it pulmonary rehabilitation.

In a pulmonary rehabilitation program, you are educated about this illness, and guided through targeted exercises that will strengthen your muscles, allowing your body to function without leaving you breathless.

And – you get to live.

Many COPD patients do not want to "make waves". The disease has a component of shame. "I did it to myself."

People are scared they will get the reception I got from that enraged doctor who told me to put my affairs in order and dramatically swept himself from the room.

They are scared that their partner will say "I told you so."

There are other causes for COPD. Chemicals, secondhand smoke. In some countries breathing the air can cause pulmonary disease. China banned junk plastic when everyone realized that was the reason they could not breathe – unregulated junk plastic refineries.

The big players in junk plastic (the plastic no one wants, single-use, not recyclable) picked up their toys and moved to Malaysia. It did not take long for villagers to develop lung disease. Malaysia has now banned junk plastic, although we still try to send it over there.

Smoking is the main contributor, though.

We have a new generation who will not go near cigarettes but are vaping their hearts out.

Sooner or later there will be an expensive inhaler with perky music ads for lung damage from vaping.

And still – a program of education and being guided through small, targeted exercise will be the most effective treatment.

COPD is also an invisible disease. People see those commercials promising that YOU CAN TAKE YOUR LIFE BACK FROM COPD! and they look at us like "What is your problem?"

Some people spend a long time pretending there is nothing wrong, until it is too late to pretend.

Even family members often do not understand what it is, to not be able to draw breath. We hear everything from "You're lazy" to "You just want to sit around and get high on oxygen."

Uh – no.

If you have someone in your life who does not get it, tell them "Clamp your nose shut. Breathe through a straw for 24 hours. Then tell me how your daily activities went."

We have the shame, the invisibility, the inhaler ads.

We have people show up on our site who are scared and confused, and do not know how to take an effective breath.

Many of them have been struggling for years. "I blow in a tube once a year and they tell me that I am going to die but I don't know when."

They have spent years looking things up on the internet, getting the Four Stages and inhaler ads. Often becoming weak, because that is what you do when you are going to die, right?

It is hard to breathe. You do not want to become breathless, so you quit moving around. The less you move, the less you want to move. You become more breathless when you move. Your muscles demand more oxygen as they get weaker. Just keeping your heart pumping can leave you breathless when you become weak.

As I said, this process of becoming weak is reversable. I was at the bottom of Stage 4, diagnosed as dead.

When Patrick told me to go to rehab, I thought he was out of his mind. I had to hold onto a wall to make it across the room.

The dogs, though. I have done many things for my dogs that I would not have done for myself.

This was the best of them.

Ongoing pulmonary rehabilitation has been nothing less than a miracle for me.

Instead of a sweaty weight room I found the essence of life itself.

We tell our people to find out if pulmonary rehabilitation is available. If they can find a rehab professional, they have struck gold.

For most, rehab is not available. If it is available, it is limited to a so many visits, or it is cost prohibitive for the patient. Or both.

Which is odd, because it is the treatment that costs the least for the medical community, put next to the inhalers and hospital stays.

Most people in rural areas have rarely even heard of pulmonary rehab. It would make sense, in a county that does not have money to toss around, to utilize a treatment that is inexpensive and effective.

The international task force recommended that legislators mandate pulmonary rehabilitation prior to or in the context of other healthcare interventions, such as expensive pharmacopeia and hospitalizations.

That would bring healthcare costs down sharply.

We are doing the opposite of that. Everyone with insurance is on at least one of the inhalers that run almost five hundred bucks a month. Often several.

The equation is simple. Pulmonary rehabilitation = longer life, increased quality of life, reduced healthcare costs.

As I said, I am not so naive that I do not know there are people happy with the expensive pharmacopeia and hospitalization cash flow.

It is time for the human cost to be taken into consideration.

It is **not** inevitable. Diagnosis, increased breathlessness, increased weakness, hospitalizations, death.

We will all die sooner or later – that part is, of course, inevitable.

The long, slow slide into the deeper stages of this disease is **not** inevitable. I am sick to death of watching my people compare inhalers, flail about blindly, and ask what a respiratory therapist does. Those without the epic good fortune to have rehab.

(Physiotherapist on Rachel's side of the pond.)

They teach you to breathe in the first few minutes they get ahold of you.

How on earth is it okay that I end up teaching some stranger to breathe when I notice she is gasping for air as she stands in line ahead of me at the pharmacy?

She told me she had been gasping for air for several years, worsening as time wore on. She was picking up an inhaler priced higher than a luxury car lease. She told me it was doing nothing for her breathing. It was making it painful to swallow and her tongue had "fuzzy white stuff" on it.

Thrush. That can end with a feeding tube. I told her to rinse and gargle with warm salt water and call her doctor immediately. No one had mentioned that, either.

She was having trouble getting a call back from her doctor.

(That is a problem many of us deal with.)

My current doctor gets back to me. He is good, as is his assistant, and the nurse practitioner I now trust. She has not once instructed me to kill myself.

When I ask her a question, she thinks, and gives me an answer. She solved the humidification dilemma with my Life2000, the only problem I had with the device. I am good to breathe now, thanks to Sossy.

The first four years of my diagnosis, I had trouble getting a call back. Except for the time they called me to tell me that I would not be scheduled for a stuffed-up nose and asked me to stop calling them.)

An inhaler will not work if you do not have the power to draw it into your lungs.

By the time she made it to the counter she was breathing through her nose, pursing her lips, and gently blowing. When she turned away from the counter and looked at me, she teared up. She told me she had forgotten what it felt like, to breathe.

Are there legislators out there willing to reduce the need for expensive pharmacopeia and hospitalizations?

Are there legislators out there not taking campaign contributions from pharmaceutical companies?

Medicare will pay for seventy-two visits. That may seem generous on the face of it. Ideally, one goes to rehab two to three times a week. It is generous, if a COPD patient wants to thrive for twenty-four weeks.

Again: Why?

Because my Decision Makers took the epic step of making ongoing pulmonary rehabilitation available, on their dime, I am living a rich life, trying to make the world around me better.

Many of us cannot work any longer.

I loved waiting tables. I was watching the news recently and saw restaurant owners talk about having a tough time finding staff. My first thought was, "It would be a great time to get a job as a waitress!"

Yeah, that would not work out. "Oxygen tube behind you!"

We contribute, though.

I am an out-of-control empath, especially with animal suffering. Once this book is out there, I will be laser-focused on animal welfare.

I usually do not advocate for humans. They have opposable thumbs.

There is a man, though, who has been imprisoned for over four decades now, despite being proven innocent. Leonard Peltier. Ten years into two life sentences they admitted prosecutorial misconduct, said they fabricated evidence, said they had no idea who killed the FBI agents Leonard was convicted of killing.

That should have been the point at which he was released. They simply changed the charges to "Aiding and Abetting".

Leonard wrote that in a very real way he died when he went to prison. He is still living out that death.

This is something that cannot stand.

I cannot change the world. Every single one of us has the power to help shape the world, though.

Ongoing pulmonary rehabilitation is the most cost-effective way to give billions of people a great shot at living their best lives.

STANDING PLACE

*M*any people consider COPD a death sentence, particularly if their lung function is low. (You are given your lung function when you perform the "Blow in the tube" test. It is also called FEV, Forced Expiratory Volume.)

Under 30% is considered "very severe". When I was diagnosed, I was at 18%. The doctor tried to put a hospital bed in my living room and call it done. Everything I Googled said that my next hospitalization would be my last.

I will be eternally grateful to Sel, who told me to quit screwing around on Facebook and find a support group, and Patrick Moan, my first Facebook doctor, who made me go to rehab.

Not only have I never been hospitalized, after two years in rehab my lung function has improved **thirty percent**, *to 24%.*

The world has closed because of the pandemic. Rehab recently opened in a limited manner – I have been able to exercise a couple of times at rehab now. Our exercise physiologist has taken me through a routine that lifts me out of tired, lifts me out of pain, brings me to a place where I feel right, living in my own skin.

When rehab closed, I got lazy and did not exercise for two weeks. I thought I was dying. Not the melodramatic "I'm gonna die!" I thought that I was moving into a deeper stage of this disease.

When I realized this, I grabbed my weights and started exercising. Immediately. Ten minutes into the routine frustration and exhaustion I did not know I had been carrying fell from my shoulders.

There will be things you cannot do any longer, and you will mourn them. Grieving is okay. Do not live there.

Find your standing place. Find what you can do, what you can have.

*Learn to **want** what you have.*

I long ago learned that gratitude heals you, emotionally.

I recently lost my partner, my support dog Tasha. She alerted when I was in respiratory distress. Friends learned to look at Tasha when they wanted to know how I was doing. She was one hundred percent focused on me, all the time. I took a shower -- the tip of her nose was inside the shower curtain.

I have grieved Tash in a way that I have never grieved anyone. I have been widowed twice. I was closer to that dog than I have been to any other living being. For years she has been within arm's reach. I fell asleep with my fingers buried in her ruff.

This has been beyond hard. I am still sitting in Tasha's dog bed. What heals me is the gratitude. I am so grateful that dog came into my life and smoothed my ragged edges. That part is permanent. Her softness has become a part of me.

I am also grateful that I had the privilege of making her last days good ones. Her first nine years were not good. Her last years were great ones. We loved each other fiercely, and the gratitude I have for that love goes deeper than pain.

*I am so rich, compared with most of the human population. So, I am attached to an oxygen tube. I **have** an oxygen tube. I have a house to put it in. All I need to do to get clean water is turn on the tap. I eat. I can provide for and protect these dogs.*

*That is **everything.***

When I was a teen I remember wandering around out there at night, seeing lit windows in houses. I wondered if I would ever have control of a light switch. It seemed out of the realm of possibility, to be able to have light whenever I wanted it.

I occasionally catch myself getting frustrated, throwing fits about something. I set a timer and allow myself to feel as sorry for myself as I can for twenty minutes. I have never made it the whole twenty minutes. It seems stupid quickly.

Taking the time to look at what is yours, and want it, will overcome just about any negative emotion you can come up with.

There are studies that are finding that gratitude heals physically, as well as emotionally.

Many of us go through life without a standing place, without even knowing that we have never had a standing place.

We react. We do what we think we are supposed to do (or not supposed to do). We reach for what we think we want, what will make us feel whole, feel better, feel different. When we get it, often it is not what we thought is would be.

So, we reach for more. We get another job. We go to school. We go through therapy. We buy a house. We sell the house. You get the picture.

We try to get by. We want to achieve something and when we do it is still not enough.

I threw drugs at my feelings. That did not work. Even at seventeen years clean and sober, though, what it was I had was not enough.

My death sentence turned out to be an enormous stroke of good fortune.

What would you do if you had a few days to live?

I had no idea what I wanted to do. I knew what I did not want. I did not want to spend my last few days on this planet feeling like I had **always** felt.

I had lived my entire life within the realm of three feelings. Scared, depressed, or loaded. I know that technically, loaded is not a feeling. It was what I aimed for when I could not stand the other ones.

My superpower of making spectacularly bad life choices had landed me in a federal penitentiary for bank robbery in the 90s. It is a long story. How to Rob a Bank in Drag. I wore heels in one of the robberies. I do not walk well on heels. The FBI analysed the tape and decided that they were after a gang of drag queens.

I am still trying to decide if I should be offended that they did not believe that women could rob banks.

I attended a five-hundred-hour drug program in prison, and cognitive therapy was thoroughly pounded into my head. I understood the principles. I believed that I was too damaged for them to apply to me.

I wiled away much of my spare time in prison listening to rock music on my Walkman and picking cognitive distortions out of rock songs.

When I was diagnosed, I stopped by the hospital to see my dad, who was dying. I then went home to meet with the people who were delivering the oxygen. While they were bustling about someone pounded on the door. I opened it, and they tried to shoulder me out of the way to move a hospital bed in my living room.

That got my attention. That doctor had told me I would not live out the week. Here was the hospital bed to prove it. I stood in front of the movers and said "Seriously? Is the guy with the rubber sheet behind you?"

I did not let them put the hospital bed in the living room. They argued with me until I finally shut the door on them. Had no one in the history of the universe ever turned down the hospital bed?

When everyone left, I sat on the floor with my dogs and my new oxygen tube. I thought, hard.

I was clean and sober. I was not going to get loaded. That left me with scared and depressed.

My fear was so huge that it went deeper than I did. It was like a separate entity. I felt like I should introduce it to people. "I'm Dawn, and this is my fear."

I could of course shut down the fear by switching over to depression. A depression so black that nothing penetrated, nothing touched me, but the dogs. The dogs got through. I felt guilty about that, though. I felt like I was depressing my dogs.

No more. I was **not** going to spend my last few days with those feelings.

I called up the cognitive therapy that had been lurking in my brain for twenty something years.

Your feelings do not come out of nowhere. They are produced by your beliefs. Challenge the belief, change the feeling. Your brain resists this for a bit, causing cognitive distortion. You pound away at it until you change the belief. Your feelings follow.

Simple. Not easy, but simple.

I spent some time alone with my dogs and tried to figure out what on earth I believed. I had no idea. Whatever it was, I had believed it since I was old enough to think.

It took some time, and some unravelling, but I got to it. I believed that I was a person-shaped piece of black ick.

I had spent my life trying to keep the black ick from leaking, trying to hide it from **everyone**.

*My first partner had told me I was secretive, that I acted like I was hiding something. I remember trying to figure out what she thought I was hiding. I have a bad habit of telling the truth about **everything** unless it involves someone else's secrets. Those I will take with me to the grave. I tell on myself all the time. I often tell people far more than they want to know.*

I had been utterly terrified, though, of someone seeing through my skin and catching a glimpse of the black ick I was made of.

I could not look people in the eye, and I did not know why.

So.

I believed I was nothing but black ick.

I looked at the evidence.

My mother was a mentally ill alcoholic, and as a child I was nourished on hatred.

I went to extreme lengths to escape her, but it appeared that I had taken the hate with me.

She sat on the top of the stairs outside my bedroom, every night. She kept a death grip on the struggling Chihuahua she was theoretically aiming her monologue at. Instead of her words, I would focus on the dog toenails scrambling across the hardwood floor as the Chihuahua tried to make a break for it, the bourbon glass hitting the floor as Mom made a grab for the Chihuahua.

The words.

*"No one wants you. No one will ever want you. I know exactly what you are up to. You are **evil**. You want to destroy my life. I can see right through you. Everyone can see right through you. You might be able to trick someone into thinking they love you some day, but they will see who you are and leave. No one will ever want you. You are evil, evil, evil"*

There were variations, but basically the same theme. Every night, for as long as I could remember. If my dad tried to shut her up, she ramped the volume way up and said she was talking to Twinkle, and it was none of his business.

Every now and again Dad would get up, take her bottle away and toss it into the street. This resulted in an uproar that had the neighbors opening their doors, and quickly closing them. Mom would become hysterical and stay that way until Dad went out in his robe to get her another bottle.

She did me a favor when I was fourteen years old. She dragged an ax up the stairs and burst into my bedroom. She was too drunk to get a good swing in, but I went to bed that night terrified. I could not help but think that I would wake up to an ax biting into my flesh.

I left the next morning. I took a paperback with me. Instead of heading for the school bus stop, I went to a Regional Transit bus stop and got on a bus that said Downtown.

(In every movie I had seen about teenage runaways, they went Downtown.)

I knew where the self-hatred came from. It was not reality. It was something that my mom had conjured.

I was not evil.

As I said, simple. Not easy.

My brain wanted to argue back. "Yes, you are evil." "No, I am not." "Yes, you are." "No, I'm not."

I kept at it until I won the argument.

Plain and simple, I was a carbon-based life form, no greater and no less than all the other carbon-based life forms out there.

We are all literally star dust.

The fear and the depression that had saturated my soul for a lifetime – lifted. It just went away.

I was left with a standing place.

I do not believe in a Higher Power. I had struggled with that for thirty-five years in a 12 Step program. That is changing, but for a long time they insisted that you must find a Higher Power of your understanding.

I tried. For thirty-five years, I tried. I prayed. I went to church. I talked to priests. Nothing. I could not feel it.

I had the long-awaited spiritual awakening and realized that, at best, I was agnostic.

*When I quit looking for a Higher Power, it freed me up to believe in **everything**. Every bright, shiny thing out there. My dog Burt's candle-glow eyes. The water catching the sunlight as a bird parties in the bird bath.*

Atoms recycle forever. There is magic in that.

When I confronted the black-ick-belief and got past it, I found out that I was worthy, and that I could take part in that magic.

I call it a lateral power. I feel connected to everything, on a deep level.

There is a bird in Delaware called the Veery thrush. A Delaware State University Professor has proved that they time their breeding season and the number of eggs they produce to leave Delaware and beat the hurricanes when they migrate to the Amazon Basin. They are so in tune with global weather patterns that they know how severe the next hurricane season will be.

They are more accurate than satellites, months before scientists start making hurricane predictions based on satellite data.

***That** is the magic of science.*

That is one example of this lateral power I have discovered that I can tap into occasionally.

I cannot predict hurricanes – that gig belongs to the Veery thrush. There are so, so many things I can celebrate, though.

I will never see most of my family again – they live on the other side of the country, and I could not take enough oxygen with me to fly there. I am not thrilled about that. I cannot even go see my kid, who is about a four-hour drive away. My portable overheats after a few hours.

I can meet with them, though. An Oculus Go Virtual Reality headset costs around three hundred dollars, a fraction of the price of a plane ticket. I can go anywhere in the world, with a 360-degree view, and meet Facebook friends there.

I watched a time-lapse of the Northern Lights and it was incredible. I did not get cold, and I did not spend all night in an airport waiting for my luggage to catch up with me.

I met Heather by a stream in Columbia. She came to live with us when she was fourteen years old and raised herself.

She looked around and said, "It looks humid."

I told her "That is what the stream is for."

People tell me "I will never see my grandkids again."

I tell them "Get a couple of Oculus Go headsets and meet up with them in Virtual Reality. You will be the cool grandparent, the one they want to spend time with." No, it is not the same as having a kid in your lap. Having a kid in your lap is not the same as having a laser sword fight and not losing your breath, though.

The standing place.

I had no idea what I wanted to do, besides live with a pack of dogs. That was a given.

I wanted to paint, but the gathering of materials and prep and cleaning up were far beyond what I could handle with my lung function.

I found a digital art class at the community college. I could do that, especially with handicapped parking a few feet away from the classroom door.

Professor Clare was incredible. She went at every student in that class and figured out how we were wired individually, how to aim teaching at us.

Drawing on the computer thrills me. The process of something emerging from nothing.

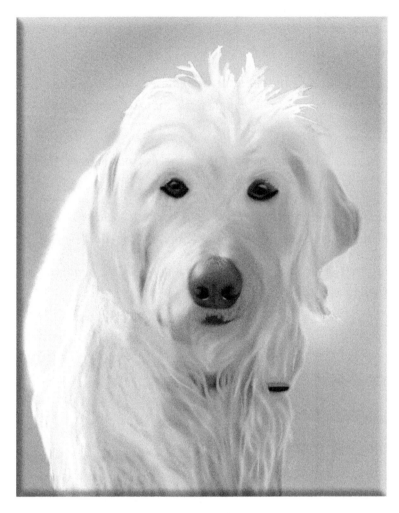

June

I take my pack to the dog park, something else I enjoy. If I pace myself and use pursed lip breathing, I have fun. Pre-rehab, it is not something I could have done.

When I am drawing a dog from the dog park, I look at them while we are visiting to see it there is anything that stands out.

I told my friend Matt that I saw June's eyelashes at the dog park.

He said "Wow. That is amazing. All that grass, and not only did you find eyelashes, you knew who they belonged to."

I lost control of an email and wrote a book.

COPD took things away. For everything is has taken, though, I have found something new to reach for.

Due to the brain fog I live with as a result of having my oxygen turned all the way up in the early years of my diagnosis, I cannot remember what I planted in the yard last year. Everything is a surprise.

Every flower is a miracle. They do not worry about what the other flowers think of them. They do not wonder if they are unfolding correctly. They do not live in terror of the bug who has its' eye on them. They unfold, and they are exquisite and perfect.

I wander around the yard saying "Wow" a lot.

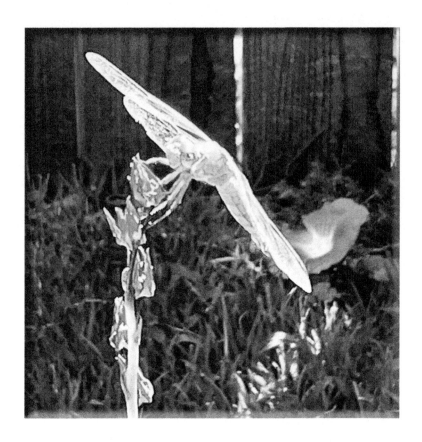

What a miracle, that I can take part in this dance.

MEDITATION AND RELAXATION

When I first met Dawn (face to face on-line) we chatted away like old friends. We then got down to business.

I asked her how she relaxes. She told me that pulling the crab grass from her garden does it for her. (It would not for me but then I hate gardening!) That is the kind of thing I get a lot when I ask patients about relaxation. They might tell me they read a book or watch a good film. And while these are perfectly good ways to spend our leisure time, it is not what I mean.

I want to know how often that person spends in a period of deep tranquility or deep relaxation. The type of relaxation where our mind is calm and settled and feelings of anxiety are reduced.

This feeling of tranquility is associated with a change in the frequency and amplitude of our brain waves (measured using an electroencephalogram (EEG).) For instance, during deep sleep (but non- dreaming) we show Delta brain wave activity. Delta waves are slow and large. As we all know deep sleep is hugely important for cell regeneration and restores us. When we are awake and active, engaged in tasks and focused, the brain waves are much faster, called Beta waves. People spend most of their waking time in Beta which uses energy and is tiring.

 Awake, we can "rest our brain" by allowing ourselves to spend periods of time in a different consciousness state.

For instance, Alpha slow waves are observed when a person is awake but resting calmly with eyes closed. But when we are deeply relaxed or meditating the brain waves slow down even further. These are known as Theta waves. Now we are in a trance like state and totally absorbed. We are curious, open to learning, to developing new behaviours and able to access the sub-conscious. We can address fears or anxieties.

It is often called a "state of wonder or awe".

It is that. I had no idea that I could go there awake. I thought the best I could hope for was that precious few second of "drifting" before I fell asleep. Rachel got me to a place where I felt like I was swinging in a hammock in my mind. Drifting, drifting, drifting…for as long as I wanted to drift.

During dreaming the brain also exhibits Theta wave activity. It is known that toddlers spend far more of their time, proportionately, in this state than in other states. That is why they can see such wonderful things!

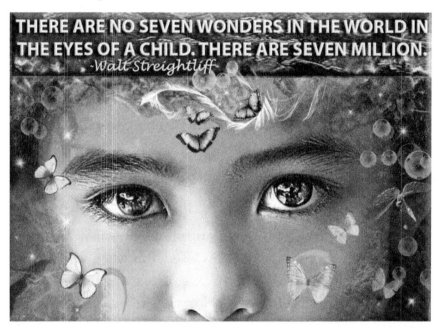

THERE ARE NO SEVEN WONDERS IN THE WORLD IN THE EYES OF A CHILD. THERE ARE SEVEN MILLION.
-Walt Streightliff

What is so special is that even as adults we can learn to gain this state of consciousness through meditation.

Scientists now know there are real long-term benefits to regular meditation, such as improvements in focus, concentration and even memory. It also has a positive effect on anxiety. In one study researchers were able to show a reduction in activity in an area of the brain called the amygdala. That is the area responsible for processing fear.

 Reductions in this area meant a reduction in anxiety for the subject.

COPD is associated with higher anxiety, cortisol and adrenalin levels. Being out of breath raises the heart rate. Learning to achieve deep relaxation is crucial. There are many guided tapes and YouTube videos available to help with this. I have made an audio tape that we you will be able to access from https://thesecrettothrivingwithcopd.com.

If you are reading a paper copy of this book and that does not turn into a link for you, go to TheSecretToThrivingWithCOPD.com. (The capitals are for the sake of readability – the internet does not care whether you use capitals or lower-case letters.)

Search YouTube. You may find others better suited to you. With trial and error, you should be able to find something that works for you. It does take practice; we recommend ten minutes daily at first, then reducing that to ten minutes four times a week when comfortable with the activity.

After our session of "Mindfulness Meditation," during which I guided Dawn into a deep relaxation, she told me she thought she had probably never totally relaxed before in her life. That is not uncommon with COPD!

I wish I could say that I stood up and lived happily ever after.

It does not work like that.

It turns out that I fall occasionally.

It is on me to ensure that I do not stay down.

It has been a tough year. We have lost three dogs and a handful of people. We tried to count and gave up.

I have heard it said a dozen different ways: The only constant in life is change.

I get to figure out how to adapt to whatever is changing, and how to keep myself together while I am trying to figure out how to adapt.

It gets confusing. When all else fails, I lay in Burt's dog bed with him.

Sel glances in and says, "You weirdo."

When we lost Peewee the entire household fell apart, each in our own way.

The house was so, so quiet. Sel asked "Did Peewee really make that much noise?"

"Yes."

Peewee had a lot to say, and she said it often.

Burt and Camden did not know what to do with themselves. I tried going to the dog park more often, but I must ration my energy. Other things I was supposed to be doing fell by the wayside.

Sel took Camden for walks to try and burn off some of her two-year-old energy. After I lost Tasha, I took in a delightful German Shepherd tripod.

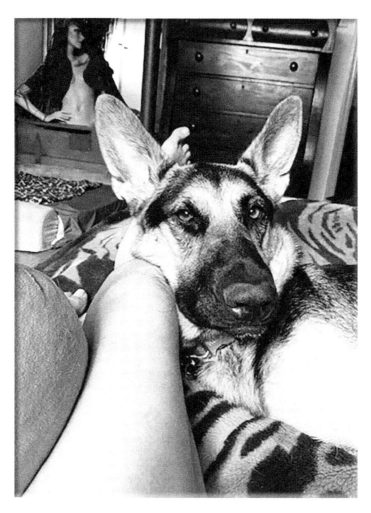

The three-legged thing does not slow Cam down a bit. She thinks that dogs with four legs are weird. She makes it work for her. She moves like a slinky at times – she can stand on her head to get her butt scratched.

Taking Camden for walks did not burn off energy. Camden did not want to go for walks. Camden wanted to go for sniffs.

She discovered a delicacy – empty snail shells.

I asked Sel "What is it called when people eat snails?"

"Escargot."

219

"Cam likes escargone!"

Camden is willful.

Sel: "Camden, get out of that bush. You are not eating those snail shells."

Camden: "Oh, I am eating those snail shells."

People walking by: "Look at that man tugging on that poor three-legged dog!"

Peewee had spent a good portion of the day chasing Camden around. Burt either hopped up and down and barked at them or chased Peewee as she chased Camden.

Without Peewee, Burt was terrified of Camden. Cam would run around tossing her toys in the air and a 96-pound Burt would land in my lap.

I do not know what the first nine years of life were for Burt.

Burt is living the dream now, but it was a year before he allowed anyone but me to touch him. He would sneak up to people and lick them. I would hear Sel in the kitchen at night.

"Whoever is licking the back of my leg stop it."

I did not go to rehab for a couple of weeks. We are going full-scale now, and every week I get a refresher on stretches from Elizabeth.

I did not want to leave the dogs alone, though. I also must admit that I had separation anxiety when I was away from my dogs.

I got depressed. I quit exercising.

Then I got scared. I started feeling like I was dying again.

I called Rick, my sponsor. I mentioned not going to rehab.

Rick said "Wait – what – whoa --..."

He was at my house the next day.

Exercising was hard at first. Again. It was not longer than two – three weeks, but it does not take long to grow weak. I had grown weak.

It took maybe a week of daily exercise, but I now feel as though I am in the process of living, not dying.

I am still getting there. Weak does not go away the second you start exercising. It is a process.

We eventually adopted a puppy. I had thought I was long past puppies, but Camden needed a running buddy. Burt, my Cowardly Lion, needed someone non-threatening.

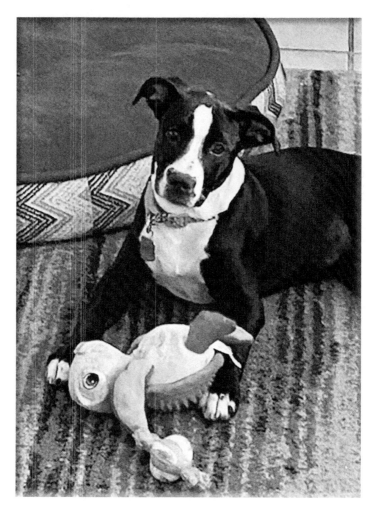

Meet Cleo.

You cannot replace a dog.

There will never be another Mojo, another Tasha, another Peewee.

Definitely not another Peewee.

When Cleo lays her head on my pillow, though, I can feel Peewee loving her with me.

I am starting to suspect that Peewee is nudging Cleo. "They really like it when you shred paper."

Peewee shredded everything. Cleo is the most well-behaved pup I have ever lived with. She goes after that paper, though.

Her foster mom told me that Cleo was not food motivated. She loves ice cubes – Cleo ice skates all over the kitchen.

Cleo's foster mom did not know the type of treats dogs get in this house. Sel cooks for them. The first time Sel stuck a piece of chicken fried steak in Burt's mouth, Burt was so stunned that he opened and closed his mouth for 20 minutes, waiting to see if it would happen again.

If it was Peewee that mentioned the paper to Cleo, she also mentioned that if you hang out politely at the edge of the kitchen when Sel cooks, you may get secret Tri-Tip. Before the official doggie Tri-Tip makes its' way around the house.

Packs evolve. Sooner or later, it will be my turn to go, and they will be looking to someone else.

In the meantime, I am grateful beyond belief for my life.

It is my job to **keep moving**, so that it is later, rather than sooner. Exercise is the most effective way to battle this disease back. Period.

I now have a puppy to outlive.

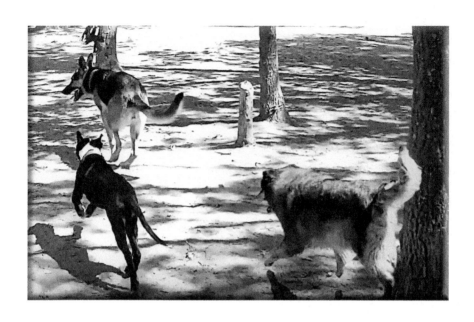

Acknowledgements

(Rachel Garrod Ph.D MSc.)

For all my patients who have taught me so much.

To Gerry, my husband, for his tolerance.

To my friends, Debbie, Hannah, Selina and Sylvia for our walks and chats. And to my constant buddy Columbus.

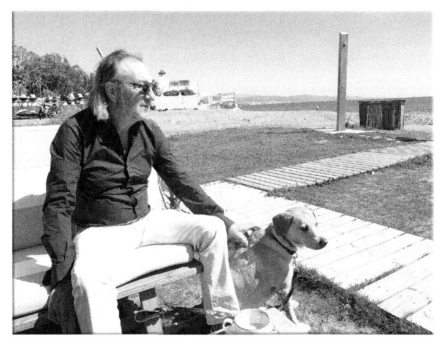

Gerry and Columbus enjoying the day.

(Dawn Lawson)

Thank you to Mark, always.

A huge thank you to Rachel Garrod. For making this book a book, for investing so much of herself in helping others, for becoming a friend.

Thank you to my friends. You know who you are, and I hope you know what you mean to me.

Thank you to my COPD group for continuing to save my life daily, especially Adele, for smiting predators while I was doing yet one more rewrite.

Thank you to Mike, Lauri, and Jeannette for your support.

Thank you to my epic Goodreads people for giving me – entertainment.

A special thank you to Dr. Angela Curiale for oh so painstakingly installing my backbone.

Thank you, Dr. Neil Flynn, Dr. David Smith, Dr. Ava Asher, and Dr. Kristen Montero for seeing me as a human being worthy of healthcare from the beginning.

Thank you, Ali, for giving me breath. Thank you, Julia, for the miracle of movement.

Thank you to my epic pulmonologist Dr. Bistrong, his assistant Drew, and equally epic nurse practitioner Sossy Farajian. Thank you to Dr. B. for designing the pulmonary rehab I attend, and for taking a chance on me by giving me a referral. A huge thank you to my healthcare system for providing pulmonary rehabilitation.

Thank you to my awesome Trilogy RT Mitch. Thank you to all the Life2000 folks at Hillrom, who respond to my every need and call just to see how I am doing. Thank you to my anonymous awesome Hillrom rep.

Thank you to Karee Rawlings, BSRC-RRT for repeatedly coming to my rescue. Thank you to my other Respiratory Care Provider, Vince Ferrara.

Thank you to the COPD Foundation for letting me pester them repeatedly, and to Pamela Denardo, COPD Coach with AARC America. Thank you to Dr. Z and the Z Pack for being healthcare professionals who are passionate about healthcare, and who have contributes to our Tricks and Hacks sheet.

Thank you to Martha Lucia for helping me find my way out of the pit known as complicated bereavement.

Finally, thank you to my pack for letting me be a boring human doing inexplicable things on a computer for lengthy periods of time.

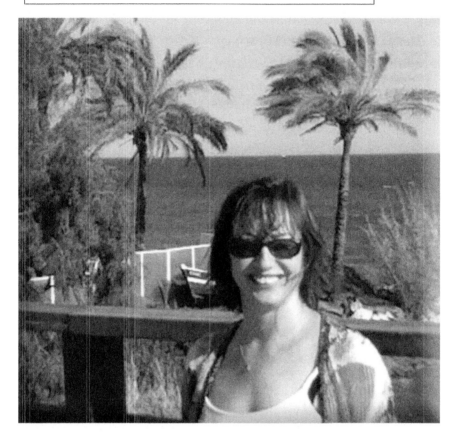

Rachel Garrod Ph.D MSc.

Rachel graduated from Guys School of Physiotherapy in 1991. Since then, she has worked in clinical practice and in academia. With over 100 peer reviewed publications, several book chapters and as editor of "Pulmonary Rehabilitation: An interdisciplinary approach". Rachel is an international expert on Chronic Obstructive Pulmonary Disease (COPD) and in Pulmonary Rehabilitation.

Rachel lives in Spain, Marbella, where she runs a private practice providing domiciliary and online respiratory physiotherapy, she runs holistic workshops on "Better Breathing" and has an online course "A Guide to Better Breathing – Physiotherapy meets Yoga."

Rachel shares her home with her husband Gerry and rescue dog Columbus. When not working, she enjoys long walks (as does Columbus, not so much Gerry,) lunches and days on the beach.

For more information about respiratory physiotherapy or to access to her course, Rachel can be contacted via email, rachelgarrod1@gmail.com, or you can join her Facebook group @PhysiotherapyforBreathingProblems.

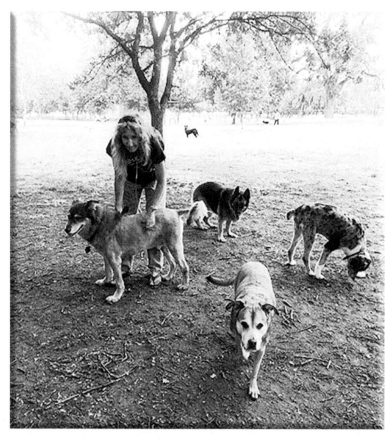

Dawn Lawson is an expert on nothing. She lives in Northern California, America, with an amazing housemate and the pack of dogs that owns them both. She is the author of HOW TO ROB A BANK IN DRAG, an autobiography, and is working on SHIMMER, a speculative fiction novel. You can follow her on goodreads.com.

Printed in Great Britain
by Amazon

15756393R00133